Monograph Book

PHARMACOLOGY OF HONEY

Editors

Dr. Narayan Dattatraya Totewad
*Department of Microbiology,
B. K. Birla College of Arts, Science & Commerce (Autonomous),
Kalyan,
Maharashtra,
India*

ABSTRACT

The antibacterial effect of honey, mostly against Gram positive bacteria, both bacteriostatic and bactericidal effects have been reported, against many strains, many of which are pathogenic. In the present research, Natural honey showed maximum Antimicrobial activity and Antioxidant activity than Commercially marketed honey. It was showed that the honey samples does not exhibited antimicrobial activity against the yeast *Candida albicans*. The pharmacological activity of Vembu honey was comparatively high when compared to the Kombu honey. All the honey samples are resistant to *Candida albicans*, *Shigella flexneri*, *Enterococcus casseliflavus* and *Pseudomonas aeruginosa*. Highest inhibitory activity was observed against *Klebsiella pneumoniae* and *Staphylococcus aureus*. In conclusion, honey is effective against the bacterial pathogens which are frequently causing Urinary tract infection and Neonatal sepsis, and it is the "SWEET MEDICINE" for bacterial infections. We also recommend the Women and Infants to take the Vembu honey regularly for preventing them from the Urinary tract infection and Neonatal sepsis.

Key words: Natural Honey, Commercial Honey, Antimicrobial activity and Antioxidant activity.

Contents

Chapter Number	Chapter Title	Page Number
1	Introduction	1
2	Review of Literature	5
3	Materials and Methods	37
4	Results and Discussion	41
5	Conclusion	56
6	References	57

1. INTRODUCTION

Microbial diseases are the major threat for the human health from the Stone Age to till now. The pathogenic activity of the microorganisms was mainly occurred due to the presence of a variety of virulence factors like capsule, endospore, antigens, polysaccharides, proteins, pili, enzymes and toxins. Among the various microorganisms in this universe, majority of the diseases are caused by bacteria and fungi. The microbial diseases are mainly transferred by three mechanisms *viz.*, Ingestion of water or food materials contaminated by microorganisms, Injection of microorganisms through insects or infected needles and Inhalation of microbial spores. In older days, the microbial infections are treated by Chemotherapy i.e., the method of treatment by using various chemicals. After the accidental discovery of the first Antibiotic Penicillin by Alexander Fleming from the mold *Penicillium notatum*, the use of chemotherapeutic agent was reduced and the peoples turned their eyes to Antibiotics. The antibiotics are the biological substance which was produced by the microorganisms which have the ability to kill or inhibit the growth of another microorganism. Based on its mode of action, antibiotics are classified into four categories *viz.*, Cell wall inhibitor, Cell membrane inhibitor, Protein synthesis inhibitor and Nucleic acid inhibitor. The first discovered antibiotic Penicillin is the Cell wall inhibitor.

After few years, the Penicillin becomes resistance to all the microorganisms and the scientists searched an alternative antibiotic for Penicillin. At the time, the great scientist who discovered more than ten antibiotics in his life time and named "Father of Antibiotics" has discovered the Protein synthesis inhibitor Streptomycin from the soil Actinobacteria *Streptomyces griseus*. The activity of Streptomycin is promising against various microbial disease and its usage was continued from previous years to present days. Nowadays, many antibiotics are commercially produced to treat various microbial diseases and it is playing an important role in the Pharmacological industry.

The antibiotic resistance has been in observed in present day against various microbial diseases due to its frequent usage. The antibiotic resistance was first observed in Penicillin against *Staphylococcus aureus* by the production of Beta – lactamase enzyme which degrades the Beta – lactum ring present in the Penicillin. But, nowadays the antibiotic resistance was extended against variety of antibiotics by many microorganisms. So, we are in need to find out an alternative medicine for treating various clinical microbial diseases caused by bacteria and fungi.

Traditional medicinal system is the method of using various natural products like seaweeds, plants and plant products for treating various diseases caused by microorganisms. The traditional medicinal system was used by the peoples in the older days but the entry of antibiotics has stopped the used of traditional medicines based treatment. The world rotation takes the peoples again to the traditional medicinal system due to the antibiotic resistance. The presence of bioactive compounds in the natural products gives an effective remedy against microbial diseases and prevents the humans from the risk of various side effects. On that line, the present study was designed to give the sweet remedy for microbial diseases using the Honey. The honey is an important part of traditional medicinal system which was used from older days to present days by all category of peoples.

The use of honey as a traditional medicine was quoted various thousands of years ago in various religious holy books like Holy Bible, Quran and Bhagavat Gita. The messenger of God, Prophet Mohammad Nabi (Peace been upon him) quoted honey as a "Healer of all diseases" Honey is a sugary syrup substance produced from the super saturated nectar, exudates of tree and secretions of plants flower by honey bees which belongs to the *Aphis* sp. it is also referred as an alimentary product of the *Aphis* sp. Biochemically, honey is composed of water and carbohydrate sugars with outstanding content of 31 % glucose and 38 % fructose and lesser content of 1 % sucrose. Honey is considered as a non-spoilage product due to the presence of mineral salts, vitamins and beneficial microorganisms. Other common ingredients of honey are amino acids (majorly proline), organic acids, hydrogen peroxide, enzymes, polyphenols, ascorbic acid, flavonoids, bee defensin, leptosin, methylglyoxal and phenolic acids. The mineral fractions available in the honey are iron, phosphorous, calcium, sodium, manganese, magnesium, copper, sodium and cobalt. Some pharmacologically important enzymes such as Glucose oxidase, Catalase, Amylase and Oxidase are present in honey (Alves Da Silva *et al.*, 2006; Saranraj *et al.*, 2016).

Nowadays, honey is considered as a "Sweet Medicine" and it does not have any medicine hatters. Honey is the product with tremendous antimicrobial activity due to the presence of phenolic compounds and it is administered orally or topically. In older days, the honey was dipped in the dressing materials and used for dressing the various types of wounds. From older days to present days, the honey was mixed with coconut oil and used for treating peptic ulcer which was caused by *Helicobacter pylori*. In human diet, honey is playing a dual role. Honey in combination with the water was used for reducing the weight and in contrast honey in combination with milk was helped to increase the weight. Initially at the time of birth, a drop of honey was given to the infants to give the sweetness and nutrients. Various researchers reported the microcidal and microstatic activities of honey samples against pathogenic bacteria and fungi. The free radical scavenging activity of honey was studied and it finds a special place as Antioxidant agent too. Honey was also used as a preservative for the preservations of various food products which are easily prone to microbial spoilage (Kalidasan *et al.*, 2017). The present study was aimed to study the comparative analysis of Antibacterial activity, Anticandidal activity and Antioxidant activity of the two Natural honey (Kombu honey and Vembu honey) and two Commercially marketed honey with following objectives.

AIM OF THE PRESENT RESEARCH

To study the Antimicrobial activity (Antibacterial and Anticandidal activity) and Antioxidant activity of Natural and Commercial honey.

OBJECTIVES OF THE PRESENT RESEARCH

1) Collection of Natural and Commercial Honey samples.
2) Determination of its Antibacterial assay.
3) Determination of its Anticandidal assay.
4) Determination of its Antioxidant activity.

2. REVIEW OF LITERATURE

With bacterial resistance to traditional antibacterial agents documented in both human and veterinary medicine, it has become necessary to investigate alternatives to commercial pharmaceuticals. Honey contains antibacterial compounds that are effective in inhibiting or killing a broad spectrum of bacteria (Bang *et al.*, 2003; Mavric *et al.*, 2008) and has been investigated as an alternative to pharmaceutical wound healing products in various parts of the world (Lotfy *et al.*, 2006; Visavadia *et al.*, 2009). A broad spectrum of antibacterial activity is valuable as many types of bacteria can pose a problem in open wounds and can impede or delay healing (Simon *et al.*, 2009). Certain plants can confer high antibacterial activity to the honey; however, there has been very little evidence to support a Canadian honey botanical source that is able to provide superior, broad spectrum antibacterial activity to honey (Brudzynski, 2006). Manuka honey, derived from the *Leptospermum* spp. plant has been shown to be antibacterial at low concentrations when compared with other types of honey (Molan, 2006).

For several decades, naturally sourced antimicrobial agents have been investigated as replacements for current pharmaceutical antimicrobials and biocides; this is increasingly the case as bacteria continue to acquire resistance to treatments (Visavadia *et al.*, 2009). These natural alternatives have been shown, in many cases, to have greater or equal efficacy when compared with other antimicrobials in tests against many species of bacteria and against multidrug resistant bacteria (Blair *et al.*, 2009). While many products have been shown to possess some antimicrobial activity, honey in particular appears to be a clinically effective antimicrobial agent. The formal discovery of the antibacterial activity in honey was made in 1892 by Dutch Scientist Van Ketel (Mohapatra *et al.*, 2011), who demonstrated that honey was capable of 'sterilizing' wounds. In human medicine, honey has been effective in treating burns, skin ulcers and other lesions (Lotfy *et al.*, 2006; Molan, 2006). A veterinary laboratory study using rabbits demonstrated that raw honey applied to open surgical wounds accelerated healing when compared to controls. Veterinary and human medical reviews have also highlighted the healing capabilities of honey in both human and animal wounds (Mathews and Binnington, 2002; Simon *et al.*, 2009).

Humans have known honey and plants for many centuries and used them as sources for nutrients as well as medicine. Today there is a growing body of literature demonstrating the efficacy of honey in various health aspects and particularly as a novel agent for wound management. The potential effects of selected honeys for the treatment of particular diseases has been known for centuries as certain honeys were selected for the treatment of particular ailments; however, it was not until recently that the research has proved that certain honeys possess unusual antimicrobial properties (Blair *et al.*, 2009) and hence have been the choice for wound management.

2.1. HISTORY OF DRUG DISCOVERY

Throughout the ages humans have relied on nature as a source of many traditional remedies and therapeutics. With the earliest Egyptian records, dating from 2400BCE, it is clear oils and plant material were utilised for their medicinal properties (David *et al.*, 2014). The Greeks and the Romans also utilised nature as a source of drug discovery (Beutler, 2009), a tradition that has been upheld through to modern medicine today as plants are the source of many nutraceuticals and pharmaceuticals (Sumner *et al.*, 2015). At the beginning of the 19th century plants were thoroughly studied to determine their therapeutic potential and during the 1970s the ocean was also targeted as a source for natural products (David *et al.*, 2014). Nearly, 50 % of the currently marketed drugs approved from 1981 to 2010 are of natural product origin (Newman and Cragg, 2012, Schmitt *et al.*, 2011). New drugs were predominantly discovered through sheer luck, inherited knowledge or trial and error up until rational drug design was developed.

Drug design starts with a hypothesis that a biological molecule may have the potential to be used as a therapeutic. Bioactive compounds have been traditionally characterized following the fractionation and purification of extracts (Sumner *et al.*, 2015). In the mid-1990s large drug companies utilised fragment based molecular modelling and computational chemistry technology to discover and produce synthetic drugs (Erlanson, 2012). The production and screening of synthetic compounds has become more accessible due to the introduction of high throughput screening methods (HTS) and modern advances in synthetic chemistry and has led to a focus on laboratory driven drug development (Cragg and Newman, 2013).

Combinatorial chemistry is a high throughput technique which has been utilized for the discovery of novel therapeutics. Points of diversity are assessed in an initial starting compound or pharmacophore. Different constructs can be created based on starting material and mathematical models (Beutler, 2009). Huge libraries can be produced and the molecular constructions can be analyzed for activity. However disadvantages include limited yield, poor solubility and low purity of the created compounds (Beutler, 2009). The success rate of drug discovery has subsequently been lower than originally expected (Newman and Cragg, 2007).

Natural product structures are not limited by the chemist's imagination and are attractive for drug discovery due to the evolution of novel bioactive secondary metabolites (Beutler, 2009). However, the use of HTS and natural products as leads for drug discovery has diminished in the past two decades (Harvey *et al.*, 2015). This trend has arisen due to the complexity of identifying, extracting and isolating new novel compounds from natural sources (Beutler, 2009). The decline or leveling out of the discovery of lead compounds by pharmaceutical companies has been evident between 1981 and 2010 (Newman and Cragg, 2012). However, natural products as a source of novel drugs are re-emerging and pharmaceutical companies are realizing that these sources need to be re-explored and combined with diversity-orientated synthetic methodologies (Newman and Cragg, 2012, David *et al.*, 2014).

Due to the significant advances in our understanding of natural-product biosynthesis, with considerable developments in approaches for natural-product isolation and synthesis new paradigms and new enterprises have recently evolved (Beutler, 2009). Transcriptomics, proteomics and metabolomics studies have recently uncovered new knowledge on biosynthesis of bioactive molecules (Sumner *et al.*, 2015, Harvey *et al.*, 2015). The production of artemisinic acid has been induced in the tobacco plant *Nicotiana benthamiana* for the treatment of malaria (Van Herpen *et al.*, 2010). The enhanced sensitivity of HTS technologies including high-performance liquid chromatography (HPLC), mass spectrometry (MS) and nuclear magnetic resonance (NMR) has advanced the ability to elucidate chemical structures from natural products (Eldridge *et al.*, 2002, Harvey *et al.*, 2015).

With the emergence of high throughput drug screening technologies related to genetic information, new lines of research are emerging to rapidly and effectively identify novel lead compounds (Singh and Barrett, 2006, Cragg and Newman, 2013). A total of 25 natural product and natural product derivatives drugs were approved for marketing from January 2008 to December 2013, 10 of these are considered to be semi-synthetic natural products and 10 were natural-product derivatives (Butler *et al.*, 2014). Surprisingly, less than 10% of the earth's biodiversity has been examined for biological activity, many more useful natural therapeutics may yet to be discovered (Harvey, 2000). By combining high throughput technology with natural product screening, nature will continue to play a vital role in the drug discovery process.

2.2. ANTIMICROBIAL NATURAL PRODUCTS

Microorganisms are common sources of novel drugs and lead compounds, which are extensively used in modern medicine (Davidson, 1995). The modern era of antimicrobial therapy began in 1929, with Fleming's accidental discovery of the bactericidal substance, penicillin (Fleming, 1929). It was observed that the growth of a fungus, from the *Penicillium* genus, had a bactericidal effect on neighboring *Staphylococcus* sp. An observation which eventually resulted in the production of many antibiotic derivatives of penicillin (Bruggink *et al.*, 1998).

The discovery of penicillin prompted increased interest in identifying novel classes of antibiotics from natural products and up till 1962 nearly all new antibiotics came from this source (Singh and Barrett, 2006). *Streptomyces* is the largest antibiotic-producing genus of bacteria, producing various antimicrobials including Streptomycin and Chloramphenicol. Antifungals including nystatin, have also been isolated from *Streptomyces noursei*. These are a few of many natural products derived from microorganisms. There is also a diverse array of unexplored potential for microbial diversity; environmental samples, extremeophiles, endophytes, marine microbes and microbial symbionts are yet to be explored (Cragg and Newman, 2013).

Evolutionarily preserved antimicrobial peptides (host defence peptides) are a diverse family of cystein-rich cationic molecules which act against a range of different microorganisms. Defensins are key elements of the innate immune response and are produced upon infection or injury to protect the host (Dossey, 2010). Naturally occurring peptides from various biological sources are utilised in modern medical therapeutics (Matsunaga *et al.*, 1985, Hopkins *et al.*, 1994, Klaudiny *et al.*, 2005).

Defensins kill bacteria by increasing the permeability of their cytoplasmic membrane resulting in a reduction of cellular cytoplasmic content (Nakajima *et al.*, 2003). Peptides have a broad antimicrobial spectrum and disrupt microbial membranes via peptide–lipid interactions by defensin oligomers. Cationic peptides interact with the negative charge of the outer membrane, disruption occurs and peptides can enter the cell. Peptides can also aggregate into the membrane forming barrel-like structures which span the membrane causing disruption of cell death (Sahl *et al.*, 2005). The inner membrane is also depolarized, cytoplasmic ATP is reduced and respiration is inhibited resulting in bacterial cell death. Three antimicrobial peptides from the marine sponge *Discodermia kiiensis*, discodermins models were among the first peptide antibiotics to be discovered and were shown to have antibacterial activity against a range of bacteria including *Pseudomonas aeruginosa*, *Escherichia coli*, *Bacillus subtilis*, and *Mycobatcerium smegmatis*.

Antimicrobial insect defensins are a large family of peptides commonly found in the hemolymph or fat cells of several insect orders, including honey bees (Ilyasov *et al.*, 2012). Honey bees produce antimicrobial defence peptides when responding to an infection (Klaudiny *et al.*, 2005). Four immune system peptides have been isolated from honey bees; apidaecin, abaecin hymenoptaecin and defensins (Casteels *et al.*, 1993). These honey bee defensins are known to leak into naturally produced bee products. Antimicrobial defensin molecules have been isolated from royal jelly (Klaudiny *et al.*, 2005, Fontana *et al.*, 2004) and more recently in Revamil® (RS) honey (Kwakman *et al.*, 2010).

2.3. EMERGING OF ANTIBIOTIC RESISTANCE IN MICROORGANISMS

The unearthing of penicillin initiated the 'Golden Age' (1940–1962) of antibiotic discovery. Many novel natural products were discovered leading to overwhelming excitement and excessive overestimations about their role in medicine (Singh and Barrett, 2006). Inappropriate and extensive use of antimicrobials in medicine, veterinary, food animal production and agriculture sectors encouraged the microorganism to mutate or acquire resistance genes, resulting in the emergence of bacterial strains with resistance to novel therapeutics (Levy and Marshall, 2004).

The mass-production and use of penicillin began in 1943 and within 4 years resistant strains of *Staphylococcus aureus* began to emerge, a trend commonly seen with many antibiotics. Methicillin resistant *Staphylococcus aureus* (MRSA), which is resistant to practically all ß-lactam antibiotics acquires resistance due to the integration of staphylococcal cassette chromosome *mec* (SCC*mec*) element. The SCC*mec* element encompasses the *mecA* gene complex and the *ccr* gene complex which encode resistance and genetic element motility and integration (Deurenberg and Stobberingh, 2008).

A report on antimicrobial resistance produced in 2014 predicts that 300 million people may die prematurely because of antimicrobial drug resistance over the next 35 years (O'Neill, 2014). The WHO reported that in the EU (and in Norway and Iceland), an estimated 25,000 people die every year because of infections related to antibiotic resistance, most of them contracted in the health care environment (WHO, 2014). These occurrences result in considerable increases in health and social costs, estimated to be € 0.9 billion annually across Europe.

The WHO global report from 2014 on surveillance of antimicrobial resistance recognizes the problems surrounding the global increase in bacterial resistance and acknowledges that MRSA is a significant threat to hospitalized and community patients (WHO, 2014). MRSA is isolated in about 5 % of all infections associated with healthcare. The WHO report (2014) highlighted that all-cause mortality, intensive care unit (ICU) mortality and bacterium-associated mortality all increase significantly with MRSA infection.

The resistance of *Escherichia coli, Neisseria gonorrhoeae* and *Klebsiella pneumoniae* to multiple drugs is on the rise (WHO, 2014). To combat this problem the WHO aim to strengthen national co-ordination and communication, to improve surveillance, to promote strategies which reduce the misuse of antimicrobials and to promote research into novel therapeutics and technologies. These strategies aim to reduce the morbidity, mortality and related expenses associated with antibiotic resistance of hospital acquired infections. Resistance management is now part of the process of identifying novel drugs as it is accepted that the emergence of resistant microorganisms is inevitable (Singh and Barrett, 2006).

2.4. FLORAL ORIGINS OF HONEY

Since the discovery of the high antimicrobial activity of manuka honey, several investigations into the floral origins and antibacterial activity of other honeys harvested globally have been reported. Identification of the floral source of honey with high antibacterial activity is important for identification of potential mechanisms of activity and for harvesting the product for medicinal use. Melissopalynological analysis (visual pollen identification) is currently the official test to determine the botanical and geographical origin of honey (Aronne and Micco, 2010). Many studies have utilized this method to determine the efficacy of honey, reporting associations between the levels of phytochemicals and antimicrobial activity by botanical source (Brady *et al.*, 2004; Irish *et al.*, 2011).

A recently reported technique for identifying the botanical origins of honey is one utilizing DNA barcoding technology, namely metagenomics. Metagenomics is a relatively new field that has been shown to be comparable to visual identification of pollen for determining the botanical origins of honey. This method is reported to be more robust, faster and simpler to implement than the classical visual methods. This method proposes a DNA barcoding approach that combines universal primers and massive parallel pyrosequencing. While this technique holds promise, further research is warranted to confirm consistent and accurate identification of floral origins of honey (Wooley *et al.*, 2010).

The introduction of honey as an effective wound care product into modern medicine has been aided by the commercialization of 'therapeutic honeys' such as manuka honey and Revamil. However, further investigation into other honeys and their floral/geographical sources is essential to determine their antimicrobial activity and their availability globally.

2.5. NOMENCLATURE AND CLASSIFICATION OF HONEY

Honey is a saturated or supersaturated sugar solution produced by social bees and some other social insects. Bees and insects gather nectar or honeydew from the flower of living plants and process by the addition of enzymes into honey, then store as a food for use in dearth periods (Crane and Visscher, 2009). Despite the contributions of few other insects honey is chiefly produced by the bees which are social insects with a perennial life cycle. The bees are mainly classified into different groups which include all honey bees (*Apis spp.*), stingless bees (*Melipona* and *Trigona* spp.) as well as *Nectarina* wasps in South America and several species of honey ants, especially *Melophorus inflatus* in Australia. There are other social wasps and bumblebees (*Bombus* spp.) with annual life cycles which produce honey, but only very little (Crane, 1999).

2.5.1. Nectar Honey

The European Commission Council Directive 2001/110/CE (EU 110, 2001) defines nectar honey as natural sweet substance produced by *Apis mellifera* bees from the nectar of plants which the bees collect, transform by combining with specific substances of their own, deposit, dehydrate, store and leave in honeycombs to ripen and mature (EU 110, 2001).

2.5.2. Honeydew honey

European Commission Council Directive 2001/110/CE defines honeydew honey as a food obtained from secretions of living parts of plants or from excretions of plant-sucking insects. The plant-sucking insects (Hemiptera) pierce the foliage or other plant covering parts, feed on the sap, and excrete the surplus as droplets of honeydew, which are gathered by the bees (EU 110, 2001). Although, the differentiation of honeydew honeys and nectar honeys could be done by pollen analysis they are far better distinguished through their physicochemical profiles since the honeydew honeys have higher pH, acidity, ash, electrical conductivity, and darker colour, as well as lower monosaccharide and a higher di- and trisaccharide content (Mateo and Bosch-Reig, 1998). In addition, honeydew contains cells of algae and fungi; however, they are not specific for its origin (Bogdanov *et al.*, 1997).

2.6. HONEY APPLICATIONS – A HISTORICAL PRESPECTIVES

Honey has been a valuable food, medicine and sweetener throughout the ages. Although it is difficult to follow exactly when the relationship between humans and the bees started and all the efforts by which ancient people have tried to domesticate the bees and how exactly humans have learned to get the best out of them this section summarizes some of the literature citing the uses of honey.

2.6.1. Honey in Ancient times

The use of honey for therapeutical purposes is well established in ancient prescriptions as well as modern wound management. The earliest records of the application of honey in medicine could be traced back to the Egyptian Papyri as well as Sumerian clay tablets dated from 1900 to 1250 BC where honey was in almost one third of the prescriptions (Molan, 1992). Other uses of honey by ancient Egyptians also included treatments for the eyes and skin as well as in embalming and wounds. "Hippocrates (460-357 BC) found that honey cleaned sores and ulcers of the lips and healed buncles and running sores. Aristotle (384-322 BC) referred to pale honey being a good salve for sore eyes" (Al Waili, 2003). The ancient Greeks were reported to have used honey to treat fatigue: athletes drank a mixture of honey and water before major athletic events (Crane, 1975).

The Babylonian used honey for the treatment of ear infections, eye infections and an ointment for the skin (Henriques, 2006). The medicinal uses of honey alone and in combination with other components including herbs and essential oils to treat various ailments including burns, wounds, eye infections as well as gastrointestinal disorders might be traced back to ancient civilizations of the Egyptians, Assyrians, Greeks and Romans (Zumla and Lulat, 1989). In 50 AD, Dioscorides described honey as being "good for all rotten and hollow ulcers" and "good for sunburn and spots on the face" (Molan, 2006). Many African tribes use honey to treat snakebites, fever and as a laxative. Moreover, the Masai warriors have used honey to gain more power and enhance their strength which is probably due to the high sugar content of honey (Henriques, 2006).

It has been reported that the Egyptians used honey in their spiced breads, cakes and pastries, and for priming beer and wine (Tannahill, 1975). In Ancient Rome honey was used in a wider range of culinary dishes. Honey has been used in salad dressings in order to balance the acidity of the vinegar as well as an essential ingredient of many sauces (Crane, 1975). Reports have mentioned that the wines drunk at the beginning and end of meals were sweetened with honey; and meat, while fruit and vegetables were sometimes preserved by immersion in honey (Free, 1982). Refined sugar which is used in cooking today has been known and used in medicines, but had no place in cooking (Wilson, 1973). Almost half of one late Roman cookery book included honey as an ingredient in almost 500 recipes (Style, 1992).

2.6.2. Honey use in Middle ages

During the Middle Ages honey was used for sweetening all type of dishes from appetizers, soups, cheese to fish dishes, roast meats as well as vegetables. However, it is difficult to predict whether a dish is savoury or sweet from the title assigned to it in a recipe. Today it is easy to predict a meat or cheese dish will usually be savoury; however, it was not the same in the Middle Ages, where meat, fish dishes and the pastry lids of 'savoury' pies might often be sweetened (Wilson, 1973).

Daude de Pradas has reported the application of honey in folk medicine in approximately 1200 AD (Crane, 1975). In a text book about honey Beck and Smedley (1997) have mentioned that honey has been used as a remedy for gastric and intestinal complaints, the diuretic effect of honey were recorded as a favoured remedy for kidney inflammations and stones. In addition Hindu people had great faith in the medical virtues of honey, mainly for the treatment of coughs, pulmonary issues and gastric disorders. Moreover, they have reported the use of particular honeys for the treatment of specific disorders and the general application of honeys for treatment of skin diseases and smallpox, as well as in surgical dressings. Furthermore, they also reported the use of a mixture of honey and crushed bees by German women for the regulation of the menstrual flow as well as the energetic and cosmetic benefits (Beck and Smedley, 1997).

2.6.3. Honey in Modern medicine

In more recent times, honey has played a relatively minor role in medicine in the developed countries mostly due to it not being accepted by Western practitioners who preferred to use to antibiotics since they were not sure of the honeys' mode of action (Molan, 1992a). However; the applications of honey continued in the Middle

East, China, Africa and Indian nations since they consider honey as a valuable source for the treatment of internal as well as external ailments (Beck and Smedley, 1997).

Populations in rural communities from almost all nations have documented the use of honey for wounds management as well as other ailments through time (Henriques *et al.,* 2010). Honey has been shown in one clinical trial to be effective against bacterial diarrhoea, (Haffejee and Moosa, 1985), and to aid in the treatment of eye infections (Molan, 2001; Al Waili, 2004). Although, honey has played a minor role in Western medicine since the development of Penicillin and other antibiotics which were considered as miracle drugs they were forced to rediscover the antibacterial potential of honeys; probably due to the emergence of multi-drug resistant pathogens such as methicillin resistant *Staphylococcus aureus* (MRSA), vancomycin resistant enterococci (VRE) and *Pseudomonas aeruginosa* (Molan, 1992).

Throughout the last two decades much research has been carried out in order to explore the mysterious role played by honey in the management of wounds and burns, which has led to scientific evidence that demonstrated honey is an effective antibacterial agent (Molan and Allen, 1996; Cooper *et al.*, 2002). The *in vitro* findings that honey is an effective antibacterial agent and proved to be even superior to many antiseptics and antibiotics are matching with the clinical trials as well as the *in vivo* and in vitro experiments that was demonstrated by many cases in which honey successfully eradicated antibiotic resistant and sensitive strains that conventional therapy has failed to eradicate (Subrahmanyam, 1991).

Medicinally, honey is used to enhance wound- healing in humans (Aysan *et al.*, 2002), treatment of gastric ulcer (Kandil *et al.,* 1987) and shortening of the duration of diarrhoea (Haffejee and Moosa, 1985). The use of honey was based on empirical knowledge rather than scientific knowledge. People didn't know how honeys cured infections but, knew it worked, this fact led to the use of antibiotics instead of honey (Molan, 2001).

Only now researchers are beginning to understand why honey has such therapeutic and beneficial potential; honey indeed could be the elixir (Molan and Allen, 1996) that the ancient people believed. Research is showing a number of other health-related benefits, including a laxative effect, beneficial effects on blood glucose levels (Cortes *et al.*, 2011), anti-inflammatory and immune stimulating properties and potentially a cancer-preventative action (Manyi-Loh *et al.*, 2011).

2.7. PRODUCTION OF HONEY

The honey bee (*Apis mellifera*) is of great importance for humans as a pollinator of both commercial and domestic crops and provider of honey, a high-value nutritional commodity (Potts *et al.*, 2010, Ratnieks and Carreck, 2010). Honey bee loss due to the interacting drivers of pests and diseases, exposure to agrochemicals, apicultural mismanagement and lack of genetic diversity have led to widespread concern about the future potential of honey bees to provide these services (Ratnieks and Carreck, 2010, Potts *et al.*, 2010). The quality and composition of honey produced is affected by many factors including flower composition, geographical position of the hive, bee health and annual changes in local flora and flowering phenology (Galimberti *et al.*, 2014). Various physical types of honey are also commercially available (comb, chunk, crystallized or granulated, creamed) with many different levels of processing (pressed, centrifuged, drained, heat processed) (Anklam, 1998).

Within a honey bee hive there are three castes – queen (alpha), worker (beta) and drone (gamma) bees (Havenhand, 2010), a collective effort allows for the production of honey. Honey is produced by honey bees using nectar from flowering plants, nectar is a sugar-rich liquid that is produced in glands called nectaries. Nectar is collected by worker bees, travelling up to 9 km in one trip (Havenhand, 2010). Sucrose in nectar is hydrolyzed to produce glucose and fructose (Kubota *et al.*, 2004). Upon return to the hive the nectar is swallowed and regurgitated by thousands of worker bees within the honey comb. The regurgitation process and wing fanning causes evaporation and the water content is reduced, the honey is ripened over time.

Honey bees keep the honey as food stores for the winter period when no nectar or pollen is available. Any excess honey can be extracted for human consumption (Havenhand, 2010). Kubota *et al.* (2004) described how glucosidase III is produced in the hypopharyngeal gland of European honey bees. This enzyme is secreted into the nectar and is responsible for the production of hydrogen peroxide (Bucekova *et al.*, 2014).

Pollen grains are collected by honey bees as they visit flowering plants to feed honey bee larvae (Galimberti *et al.*, 2014). Dense pollen pellets are produced from these grains using a nectar-saliva mixture. Honey bees collect the exudate from sap-sucking insects as an alternative to nectar. Honeydew collection is often recorded from sap feeding insects feeding on conifers and other anemophilous species (Oddo *et al.*, 2004). Tree resin is also actively collected from a range of species and combined with wax to make propolis that is deposited within the hive as it has antimicrobial properties (Wilson *et al.*, 2013).

2.8. COMPOSITION OF HONEY

Honey contains an array of minor constituents including carbohydrates, volatiles and phenolic compounds including flavonoids and non-flavonoid phenolic compounds (Baroni *et al.*, 2006). These compounds originate from plants foraged upon by the bees and from the bees themselves. Phenolic compounds are affected by the storage and processing of the honey, microbial or environmental contamination, geographical distribution and botanical source of nectar and pollen. Although, honey is a unique saturated complex solution all honeys are not the same since they vary depending on the variation in their botanical source, geographical location, bee species, storage condition, beekeeping as well as the year and time of collection during the year all could affect the chemical profile of the honey (Manyi-Loh *et al.*, 2011).

2.8.1. Osmalarity

Due to the high sugar content of honey, the osmotic pressure of honey is usually high leading to low water activity (a_w) reported range = 0.562 – 0.62 (Bogdanov *et al.*, 1997), which gives the osmolarity an essential role in the antimicrobial activity of undiluted honeys; since, the growth of many bacterial species, for example, is completely inhibited when the (a_w) is in the range of 0.94 - 0.99 (Molan, 1992).

2.8.2. Water content

Honey water content is an important quality parameter, which must be determined in order to prevent the spoilage of honey due to fermentation. The honey moisture content is not like other parameters which are optionally accepted, since it affects the quality as well as the shelf life of the honey (Bogdanov *et al.*, 2004). The International Honey Commission (IHC) has set a maximum limit of 20g water/100g of honey for any honey sample to be accepted for honey trade. The moisture content has a direct effect on other honey properties such as glucose crystallization and viscosity of the honey (Bogdanov *et al.*, 2004). The honey moisture content is evaluated by either refractive index, gravimetric technique or Karl Fischer titration (Sanchez *et al.*, 2010).

2.8.3. Acidity

Acidity is another factor which contributes to the antimicrobial activity of honey. Although it was thought to have a major role, more recent studies have demonstrated that acidity actually plays a minor role in the antibacterial activity of honey (Molan, 1992). There are about 30 organic acids in honey (Mato *et al.*, 2003); however, gluconic acid which is produced due to the activity the enzyme glucose oxidase is main organic acid present in the honey in the range of 0.23 - 0.98 % (White, 1975).

2.8.4. Sugar content (Carbohydrates)

Honey is a complex saturated or super saturated solution which mainly made up of two components sugars and water. The sugars or carbohydrates make up more than 90 % of the honey's total dry matter (Anklam, 1998). It has been reported that honey is made up of more than 180 substances (Jones, 2009) which Bogdanov has estimated to be actually even closer to 600 substances (Bogdanov *et al.*, 2004). The carbohydrates content of honeys includes a variety of sugars such as the monosaccharides fructose (levulose) as well as glucose (dextrose), sucrose and maltose and disaccharides oligosaccharides which seem to differ according to the floral source of the honey (Molan and Allen, 1996).

Sugars (saccharides) comprise the major portion of honey approximately 85 - 95 % (w/v) of the total honey. Honey consists mostly of the monosaccharides fructose and glucose. Twenty five other oligosaccharides (disaccharides, trisaccharides, tetrasaccharides) have also been described. Invert syrup (IS), conventional corn syrup (CCS) and high fructose corn syrup (HFCS) is also used in honey adulteration (Anklam, 1998). Honey is a variable and complex mixture of sugars and other components.

At its very basic level, honey consists of a mixture of simple carbohydrates which create a highly osmotic environment. The combination of low levels of water (~18 %) and high levels of sugar (~80 %) are enough in themselves to prevent the spoilage of honey by microorganisms (Kwakman *et al.*, 2010). Disruption of the bacterial cell wall occurs due to the osmotic effect. The osmotic effect has been shown to be an important parameter for killing *Helicobacter pylori*, however honey has other antibacterial factors beyond the osmotic effect (Kwakman and Zaat, 2012). An artificial honey solution is used to distinguish between the osmotic effects of sugars and antibacterial activity in a study by Cooper *et al.* (2002).

2.8.5. Proteins and Amino acids

Honey normally contains between 0.1 - 0.5 % protein (Won *et al.*, 2009). Eighteen amino acids are found in honey; proline represents 50 – 85 % of the total amino acid profile. Arginine, tryptophan, and cystine are characteristic amino acids in some honey types (Anklam, 1998). Enzymes make up a small fraction of these proteins. Enzymes found in honey which originate from both nectar and the bees are common (Weston, 2000). Predominant enzymes are diastase (amylase), which breaks down starch into smaller units; invertase (glucosidase) which converts glucose to fructose and glucose oxidase which catalyses the reaction of glucose to gluconolactone, resulting in the production of gluconic acid and hydrogen peroxide (Bucekova *et al.*, 2014). Catalase occurs naturally in some pollen grains, catalase neutralizes hydrogen peroxide (Assia and Ali, 2015).

2.8.6. Vitamins and Minerals

Trace amounts of B vitamins (riboflavin, niacin, folic acid, pantothenic acid and vitamin B6) and C vitamins (ascorbic acid) are found in honey. Many different minerals (calcium, iron, zinc, potassium, chromium, phosphorous, magnesium and manganese) are found in unprocessed honey.

2.8.7. Volatile compounds

More than 600 volatile organic compounds (VOCs) have been identified in honey. Volatiles are organic chemicals that have a high vapour pressure at standard room temperature. Seven major groups have been previously characterised in honey; aldehydes, ketones, acids, alcohols, esters, hydrocarbons and cyclic compounds (Kaskonienė and Venskutonis, 2010; Manyi-Loh *et al.*, 2011).

Honey contains numerous VOCs in low concentration however, VOCs affect the sensory characteristic of honey; flavour, aroma, colour and texture are all effected by the type of plants and flowers bees visit (Manyi-Loh *et al.*, 2011). Some VOCs originate from the plants or nectar source whereas others are created during the processing or storage of honey (Jerkovic *et al.*, 2006, Castro-Vazquez *et al.*, 2008; Jerkovic *et al.*, 2011). The Maillard reaction occurs when honey is heat treated; a non-enzymatic browning reaction occurs between sugars and amino acids resulting in the production or transformation of VOCs (Castro - Vazquez et al., 2008). Microbial and environmental contamination can also contribute to the number of VOCs (Manyi - Loh et al., 2011).

2.8.8. Hydroxymethylfurfuraldehyde (HMF)

Hydroxymethylfurfuraldehyde (HMF) is also present in minor quantities. HMF which could be formed in the presence of acid due the breakdown of fructose has been considered as evidence for the adulteration of honey; however, it has been proved that even fresh honeys do contain minor amounts of HMF (Zappala et al., 2005) which could easily be elevated if the honey is stored in moderate or high temperatures; hence, it is necessary to store honey in a refrigerator or a cool place (White, 1975) so as to keep the levels of HMF to the minimum since, HMF is one of the main factors which are considered for the quality and marketing of honey.

2.8.9. Enzymes

Moreover, honey contains a number of enzymes including glucose oxidase, invertase, and amylase, which appear to originate from honeybees (Molan, 1992). Glucose oxidase plays an essential role in the antibacterial activity of honeys as well as the generation of gluconic acid. The enzyme Invertase catalyses the conversion of sucrose obtained from the nectar and into the monosaccharides fructose and glucose in a ratio of 1.2:1 between glucose and fructose (Anklam, 1998). There are other enzymes such as catalase and acid phosphatase (White, 1975) which are also present in some honeys but these are likely to be derived from the pollens and nectar of plants.

2.8.10. Phenolic compounds

The major phenolic compounds identified in honey are flavonoids: quercetin, pinocembrin, pinobanksin, chrysin, galangin, kaempferol and luteolin (Pyrzynska and Biesaga, 2009; Kaskonienė and Venskutonis, 2010; Dong et al., 2013). Aromatic acids contain an aromatic ring and an organic acid function (C6-C1 skeleton). Phenolic compounds are an example of aromatic acids as they containing a phenolic ring and an organic carboxylic acid function. Phenolic acids can be found in many plant species (Cai *et al.*, 2004; Lin and Harnly, 2007; Pinho *et al.*, 2014). Flavonoids are plant specialized metabolites which fulfil many functions and are important for plant pigmentation, UV filtration and symbiotic nitrogen fixation (Dixon and Pasinetti, 2010). Flavonoids are widely distributed in plants and their basic molecular structure is 2-phenyl-1,4-benzopyrone. Plant derived phenolic acids include benzoic, ferulic, gallic, chlorogenic, caffeic, p-coumaric, ellagic and syringic acids. Phenolic compounds have antibacterial, anti-inflammatory and antioxidant activities. The composition of phytochemicals has an effect on the bioactivity of honey (Kaskonienė and Venskutonis, 2010).

2.8.11. Pollen, Proposils and Royal jelly

Honey bees collect pollen and nectar from flowering plants, supplying the hive with protein for nourishment. Pollen is commonly found in honey. Wind pollinated pollen from trees and plants also frequently feature within honey (Bruni *et al.*, 2015). Pollen contains contain carbohydrates, amino acids, DNA, nucleic acids, proteins, lipids, vitamins, minerals, phenolic compounds and flavonoids (Morais *et al.*, 2011).

Propolis is produced from the exudates of plants; bees seal the hive with the resinous substance creating a protective barrier against intruders (Viuda - Martos *et al.*, 2008). Propolis is comprised of resin (50 %), wax (30 %), essential oils (10 %), pollen (5 %), and other organic compounds (5 %) (Viuda - Martos *et al.*, 2008). More than 300 compounds including phenolic compounds, esters, flavonoids, terpenes and anthraquinones have been found in propolis (Kalogeropoulos *et al.*, 2009, Bertrams *et al.*, 2013).

Royal jelly is a proteinous liquid secreted by glands in the hypopharynx of worker bees; it is produced exclusively for the adult queen bees, it is a vital nutritional source (Viuda - Martos *et al.*, 2008). More than 50 % of the dry mass of royal jelly is proteins, major royal jelly proteins (MRJPs) have been researched and analysed (Won *et al.*, 2009). Royal jelly is used as a dietary supplement for the treatment of many conditions including asthma, high cholesterol and seasonal allergies.

2.8.12. Hydrogen peroxide

In the 1960s, hydrogen peroxide (H_2O_2) was identified as a major antibacterial compound in honey. Hydrogen peroxide is commonly used in cleaning products such as bleach but it is also produced naturally during glucose oxidation of honey (Brudzynski *et al.*, 2011). Hydrogen peroxide is also a contributing factor to a honeys acidity and sterility.

Hydrogen peroxide and honey phenolics with pro-oxidant activities are involved in oxidative damage resulting in bacterial growth inhibition and DNA degradation (Brudzynski *et al.*, 2011, Brudzynski *et al.*, 2012). Brudzynski *et al.* (2012) concluded that hydrogen peroxide is involved in oxidative damage, which causes bacterial DNA degradation and growth inhibition. Further studies revealed the bacteriostatic effect was directly related to the generation, and therefore concentration of hydroxyl radicals generated from the hydrogen peroxide (Brudzynski and Lannigan, 2012). It is believed that the hydrogen peroxide effects are modulated by other honey components (Brudzynski *et al.*, 2011).

2.8.13. Bee derived antimicrobial peptides

Bee derived defensins are cysteine-rich cationic peptides produced in the salivary glands and fat body cells and are involved in social and individual immunity (Klaudiny *et al.*, 2005). Two defensins have been characterised, royalisin (from royal jelly) and defensin (from the haemolymph), which are both encoded by Defensin - 1. The Defensin - 2 which shows 55 % similarity to Defensin - 1, has also been identified (Ilyasov *et al.*, 2013). Defensin-1 (5.5 KDa) has been shown to possess potent antibacterial activity against Gram positive microorganisms including *Staphylococcus aureus* and *Bacillus subtilis* (Kwakman *et al.*, 2010; Bucekova *et al.*, 2014) and *Paenibacillus* larvae. This is the causative agent of American Foulbrood (AFB) which is a major pathogen of bees (Katarina *et al.*, 2002).

The honey is not registered as an antimicrobial but as a wound healing stimulant where it is claimed to stimulate tissue regeneration and reduce inflammation. The *in vitro* bactericidal activity against *Bacillus subtilis*, *Staphylococcus aureus*, *Streptococcus epidermidis*, *Escherichia coli* and *Pseudomonas aeruginosa* was assessed and a bactericidal effect was seen within 24 hrs by 10 - 40 % (v/v) honey (Kwakman *et al.*, 2010). The peptide (defensin-1) and the other factors contributing to this bactericidal effect were also characterized (Kwakman *et al.*, 2010). Other proteinaceous antibacterial compounds have previously been reported in six of twenty six honeys, but identification of these proteins was not performed (Mundo *et al.*, 2004).

2.8.14. Plant derived antimicrobial phytochemicals

Plant derived phytochemicals play an important role in the antibacterial activity of honey; methylglyoxal (MGO) from Manuka honey is an example of honey which attributes its activity to plant derived chemicals. Non-peroxide activity has been described in investigations of bactericidal factors within honey (Manyi-Loh *et al.*, 2012; Pinho *et al.*, 2014), particular attention has been paid to Manuka honey (Adams *et al.*, 2009).

Plant derived phenolic compounds isolated from honey have been investigated and identified by different research groups, but the contribution to the overall activity remains unclear (Isla *et al.*, 2011; Manyi-Loh *et al.*, 2012; Kwakman and Zaat, 2012; Liu *et al.*, 2013) It has been suggested that the contribution of plant derived components to the antibacterial activity of honey is too low to detect (Kwakman *et al.*, 2010), but when extracted phenolics and flavonoids are regarded as a very promising source of natural medicinal therapeutics.

Solid phase extraction (SPE) and HPLC analysis was used to extract phenolic compounds and antimicrobial agents from *Rubus* honey (Escuredo *et al.*, 2012). The phenolics caffeic, *p*-coumaric and ellagic acids and the flavonoids chrysin, galangin, pinocembrin, kaempferol and tectochrysin were isolated (Escuredo *et al.*, 2012). The phenolic fraction samples showed antimicrobial activity against various organisms including *Salmonella typhimurium*, *Proteus mirabilis* and *Pseudomonas aeruginosa*. The most susceptible species were *Proteus mirabilis* and *Bacillus cereus* (Escuredo *et al.*, 2012). The antioxidant and antimicrobial activities of phenolics extracted from *Rhododendron* honeys from the Black Sea region of Turkey have also been studied (Silici *et al.*, 2010). High levels of antimicrobial activity were described against *Pseudomonas aeruginosa* and *Proteus mirabilis* (Silici *et al.*, 2010). The combination of different phenolics, instead of individual compounds may contribute to the activity of honey, but further investigations are required in order to assess these interactions (Manyi - Loh *et al.*, 2012). The minor constituents in honey have high levels of antimicrobial activity due to a combination of these factors, often working in unison. These plant derived compounds have high potential to be used as therapeutics in human health.

It has been shown that the flavonoids, phenolic and organic acids in honey may act in various processes including hydrogen donating, oxygen quenching, radical scavenging and metal ion chelation resulting in bacterial growth inhibition (Manyi - Loh *et al.*, 2012). The antibacterial activity of phenolic compounds should not be dismissed; phytochemicals have an influence on the antimicrobial activity of honey (Molan, 2011). Peroxide and non-peroxide factors may also be working in synergy and inhibiting bacterial growth (Manyi-Loh *et al.*, 2011).

In order to analyze these compounds, the sugars which are the major components in honey must be removed. Various analytical techniques can be used to identify these components (Cuevas-Glory *et al.*, 2007, Pontes *et al.*, 2007). Thin Layer Chromatography (TLC) and Gas Chromatography-Mass Spectrometry (GC-MS) have been used to extract the phenolic compounds which have demonstrated antibacterial activity against *Helicobacter pylori* (Manyi-Loh *et al.*, 2012). The *Helicobacter pylori*, which cause chronic active gastritis and peptic ulcers, showed susceptibility to various fractions of South African honey (Manyi - Loh *et al.*, 2012; Manyi - Loh *et al.*, 2013). The activity was attributed to the combination or separate action of volatile compounds including acetic acid (Manyi - Loh *et al.*, 2012).

Other VOCs have been identified in honey; (±)-3-Hydroxy-4-phenyl-2-butanone and (+)-8-hydroxylinalool show high levels of antimicrobial activity against bacteria including *Staphylococcus aureus, Escherichia coli, Klebsiella pneumoniae* and human pathogen fungi *Candida albicans* (Melliou and Chinou, 2011). Despite only being present in low concentrations the VOCs may contribute to the overall antimicrobial activity and have the potential to be used as natural therapeutics to treat a range of pathogenic microbial organisms.

2.8.15. Other minor components

Furthermore, honey is rich with other components although in minor amount. These include amino acids (mainly proline), vitamins including vitamin A, B-vitamins (riboflavin, niacin, pyridoxine, panthothenic acid, and folic acid), vitamin-C (ascorbic acid), vitamin D, and vitamin E, Honey also contains a significant number of minerals, including calcium, phosphorous, iron, zinc, selenium, chromium, potassium, magnesium, and manganese, and organic acids (Bobis *et al*, 2008). Other components present in honeys also include flavonoids, antioxidant substances and unidentified plant-derived elements (phytochemical components) (Sato and Miyata 2000).

2.9. ANTIMICROBIAL EFFICIENCY OF HONEY

The antibacterial effect of honey, mostly against Gram positive bacteria, both bacteriostatic and bactericidal effects have been reported, against many strains, many of which are pathogenic. Honey glucose oxidase produces the antibacterial agent hydrogen peroxide, while another enzyme, catalase breaks it down. Honey with a high catalase activity has a low antibacterial peroxide activity. Honey has both peroxide and non peroxide antibacterial action, with different non-peroxide antibacterial substances involved: acidic, basic or neutral (Bogdanov, 2006).

Antimicrobial effect of honey is thus due to different substances e.g. aromatic acids and compounds with different chemical properties and depends on the botanical origin of honey. The high sugar concentration of honey, and also the low honey pH is also responsible for the antibacterial activity. Most experiments report on stop of bacterial growth after a certain time of honey action. The higher the concentration the longer is the period of growth inhibition. Complete inhibition of growth is important for controlling infections. Honey has also antiviral activity Rubella, Herpes virus (Al-Waili, 2004).

Honey has also fungicide activity against different dermatophytes. Honey has been shown to have a prebiotic effect, i.e. its ingestion stimulates the growth of healthy specific Bifidus and *Lactobacillus* bacteria in the gut. Sour-wood, alfalfa, sage and clover honeys have been shown to have prebiotic activity. The prebiotic activity of chestnut honey is bigger than that of acacia honey. Oligosaccharides from honeydew honey have prebiotic activity. Theoretically honeydew honeys, containing more oligosaccharides should have a stronger prebiotic activity than blossom honeys (Stefan Bogdanov, 2011).

2.9.1. Antibacterial activity

The antibacterial properties of honey includes, the release of low lives of hydrogen peroxide, some honey have an additional phytochemical antibacterial compounds. The antibacterial property of honey is also due to osmotic effect of its high sugar content as it has an osmolarity sufficient to inhibit the microbial growth (Rakhi *et al.*, 2010). Hydrogen peroxide was responsible for the antibacterial activity of honey since both the antibacterial activity of honey and hydrogen peroxide were destroyed by light (Miki Fukuda, 2011). White and Subers reported that hydrogen peroxidase which is produced by the glucose oxidase of honey could be the inhibitory substance against bacteria. However, it is known that honey as well as bacteria produces a catalase that eliminates hydrogen peroxide. But although catalase is active with high concentration of hydrogen peroxide, it is of low activity with physiological levels (Osho and Bello, 2010). Lavie found an additional group of light sensitive, heat-stable antibacterial factors in honey which inhibited the growth of *Bacillus subtilis*, *Bacillus alvei*, *Escherichia coli*, *Pseudomonas pyocyanes*, *Salmonella typhi* and *Staphylococcus aureus* (Laid Boukraa, 2008).

A comparison was made by Cortopassi – Laurino and Gelli between the physico-chemical properties and antibacterial activity of honey produced by Africanized honey bees (*Aphis mellifera*) and Melliponinae (stingless bees) in Brasil. For both types of honey at a concentration of 5 – 25 %, *Bacillus stearothermophilus* was found to be the most susceptible and *Escherichia coli* the least susceptible of the seven bacterial isolates tested (the other five being, *Bacillus subtilis, Staphylococcus aureus, Klebsiella pneumoniae* and *Pseudomonas aeruginosa*). *Melipona subnitida* honey produced from *Mimosa bimucronata* and *Plebia* sp. honey produced from *Borreria/Mimosa* exhibited the greatest antibacterial activities (White and Subers, 2013).

Antibacterial activities of the two honey samples, produced by the honeybee (*Aphis mellifera*), were assayed using standard Well diffusion method. Both honey samples were tested at four concentrations (5 %, 25 %, 50 % and 100 % w/v) against *Staphylococcus aureus, Pseudomonas aeruginosa, Klebsiella pneumoniae, Bacillus subtilis* and *Escherichia coli*. There are many reports of bactericidal as well as bacteriostatic activity of honey and the antibacterial properties of honey may be particularly useful against bacteria, which have developed resistance to many antibiotics (Osho and Bello, 2010).

2.9.2. Antifungal activity

The synergistic action of starch on the antifungal activity of honey, a comparative
method of adding honey with and without starch to culture media was used. *Candida albicans* has been used to determine the minimum inhibitory concentration (MIC) of five varieties of honey (Conti, 2000). The antifungal action of three single samples of South African honey (wasbessie, bluegum and fynbos) against *Candida albicans* and found honey to inhibit on the growth of *Candida albicans*, while the control, bluegum and fynbos honey produced only partial inhibition (Terrab *et al.*, 2004).

2.9.3. Antiviral activity

Honey had good anti-Rubella activity, while thyme did not. These results may justify the continuing use of honey in traditional medicines from different ethnic communities worldwide and in some modem medications such as cough syrups (Golob et al., 2005).

2.10. ANTIOXIDANT ACTIVITY OF HONEY

Honey contains a variety of phytochemicals (as well as other substances such as organic acids, vitamins, and enzymes) that may serve as sources of dietary antioxidants (Gheldof and Engeseth, 2002). The amount and type of these antioxidant compounds depends largely upon the floral source/variety of the honey. In general, darker honeys have been shown to be higher in antioxidant content than lighter honeys. Researchers at the University of Illinois Champaign/Urbana examined the antioxidant content (using an assessment technique known as Oxygen Radical Absorbance Capacity or ORAC) of 14 unifloral honeys compared to a sugar analogue. ORAC values for the honeys ranged from 3.0 μ mol TE/g for acacia honey to 17.0 μ mol TE/g for Illinois buckwheat honey.
The sugar analogue displayed no antioxidant activity (Swellam et al., 2013).

Free radicals and reactive oxygen species (ROS) have been implicated in contributing to the processes of aging and disease. Humans protect themselves from these damaging compounds, in part, by absorbing antioxidants from high-antioxidant foods. This report describes the effects of consuming 1.5 g/kg body weight of corn syrup or buckwheat honey on the antioxidant and reducing capacities of plasma in healthy human adults. It can be speculated that these compounds may augment defenses against oxidative stress and that they might be able to protect humans from oxidative stress. Given that the average sweetener intake by humans is estimated to be in excess of 70 kg
per year, the substitution of honey in some foods for traditional sweeteners could result in an enhanced antioxidant defense system in healthy adults (Derek et al., 2013).

Antioxidant properties shown by volatile oil of propolis (VOP) from India were investigated by spectrophotometric methods and a photochemiluminescence method and it was found that from IC50 values it could be concluded that the efficiency of scavenging ABTS radicals by the VOP was more pronounced as compared to scavenging other radicals (Orsolic *et al.*, 2013).

2.11. OTHER MEDICINAL USES OF HONEY
2.11.1. Honey as Antibiotics

Manuka honey has potent antibacterial properties, making it especially beneficial for preventing and treating wound infections by drug-resistant bacteria, according to physician Robert Frykberg of the Veterans Affairs Medical Center in Phoenix, Ariz.

2.11.2. Antidiabetic activity

Frykberg noted that the FDA-approved manuka honey product, Medihoney, has proven beneficial for healing foot ulcers in diabetic patients. Diabetics with foot ulcers that do not heal sometimes require foot amputation.

2.11.3. Arthritis

Take one part honey to two parts of luke warm water and add a small teaspoon of cinnamon powder, make a paste and massage it on the itching part of the body. It is noticed that the pain recedes within a minute or two. Or for arthritis patients daily morning and night take one cup of hot water with two spoons of honey and one small teaspoon of cinnamon powder. If drunk regularly even chronic arthritis can be cured. In a recent research done at the Coppen Hagen University, it was found that when the doctors treated their patients with a mixture of one tablespoon honey and half teaspoon cinnamon powder before breakfast, they found that within a week out of the 200 people so treated practically 73 patients were totally relieved of pain and within a month, mostly all the patients who could not walk or move around because of arthritis started walking without pain.

2.11.4. Hair Loss

Those suffering from hair loss or baldness may apply a paste of hot olive oil, one tablespoon or honey, one teaspoon cinnamon powder before bath and keep it for approximately 15 min. And then wash the hair. It was found very effective even if kept for 5 min.

2.11.5. Bladder Infections

Take two tablespoons of cinnamon powder and one teaspoon of honey in a glass of luke warm water and drink it. It destroys the germs of the bladder.

2.11.6. Toothache

Make a paste of one teaspoon of cinnamon powder and five teaspoons of honey and apply on the aching tooth. This may be done 3 times a day daily till such time that the tooth has stopped aching.

2.11.7. Cholesterol

Two tablespoons of honey and three teaspoons of cinnamon powder mixed in 16 ounces of tea water if given to a cholesterol patient; it reduces the level of cholesterol in the body by 10 % within 2 hours. As mentioned for arthritic patients, if taken 3 times a day any chronic cholesterol cured. As per the information received in the said journal, pure honey taken with food daily relieves complains of cholesterol.

2.11.8. Colds

Those suffering from common or severe colds should take one tablespoon Luke warm honey with 1/4 teaspoon cinnamon powder daily for 3 days. This process will cure most chronic cough, cold and clear the sinuses.

2.11.9. Stomach upset

Honey taken with cinnamon powder cures stomachache and also clears stomach ulcers from the root. Gas: according to the studies done in India and Japan, it is revealed that if honey is taken with cinnamon powder the stomach is relieved of gas.

2.11.10. Heart Diseases

Make a paste of honey and cinnamon powder, apply on bread or chapatti instead of jelly and jam and eat it regularly for breakfast. It reduces the cholesterol in the arteries and saves the patient from heart attack. Also those who have already had an attack, if they do this process daily, are kept miles away from the next attack, regular use of the above process relieves loss of breath and strengthens the heart beat in America and Canada, various nursing homes have treated patients successfully and have found that due to the increasing age the arteries and veins, which lose their flexibility and get clogged, are revitalized.

2.11.11. Immune system

Daily use of honey and cinnamon powder strengthens the immune system and protects the body from bacterial and viral attacks. Scientists have found that honey has
various vitamins and iron in large amounts. Constants use of honey strengthens the white
blood corpuscles to fight bacterial and viral diseases.

2.11.12. Indigestion

Cinnamon powder sprinkled on two tablespoons of honey taken before food, relieves acidity and digests the heaviest of meals.

2.11.13. Influenza

A scientist in Spain has proved that honey contains a natural ingredient, which kills the influenza germs and saves the patient from flu.

2.11.14. Longevity

Tea made with honey and cinnamon powder, when taken regularly arrests the ravages of old age. Take 4 spoons of honey 1 spoon of cinnamon powder and 3 cups of water and boil to make like tea. Drink 1/4 cup, 3 to 4 times a day. It keeps the skin fresh and soft and arrests old age. Life spans also increases and even if a person is 100 years old. Starts performing the chores of 20 years old.

2.11.15. Pimples

Three tablespoons of honey and one teaspoon of cinnamon powder paste. Apply this paste on the pimples before sleeping and wash it next morning with warm water. If done daily for two weeks. It removes pimples from the roots.

2.11.16. Skin infections

Applying honey and cinnamon powder in equal parts on the affected parts cures eczema, ringworm and all types of skin infections.

2.11.17. Weight loss

Daily in the morning 1/2 hour before breakfast on an empty stomach and at night before sleeping, drink honey and cinnamon powder boiled in one cup water. If taken regularly it reduces the weight of even the most obese person. Also drinking of this mixture regularly does not allow the fat to accumulate in the body even though the person may eat a high calorie diet.

2.11.18. Cancer

Recent research in Japan and Australia has revealed that advanced cancer of the
stomach and bones have been cured successfully. Patients suffering from these kinds of
cancer should daily take one tablespoon of honey with one teaspoon of cinnamon powder for one month 3 times a day.

2.11.19. Fatigue

Recent studies have shown that the sugar content of honey is more helpful than detrimental to the body strength. Senior citizens who take honey and cinnamon powder in equal parts are more alert and flexible. Dr. Milton who has done research says that half tablespoon honey taken in one glass of water and sprinkled with cinnamon powder, taken daily after brushing and in the afternoon at about 3:00 p.m.

When the vitality of the body starts decreasing. Increases the vitality of the body within a week.

2.11.20. Bad breath

People of South America, first thing in the morning gargle with one teaspoon of honey and cinnamon powder mixed in hot water. So, their breath stays fresh throughout the day.

2.11.21. Hearing loss

Daily morning and night honey and cinnamon powder taken in equal parts restores hearing.

2.11.22. Wound Healing

Honey is one of the oldest known medicines that have continued to be used up to present times in folk-medicine. Its use has been "rediscovered" in later times by the medical profession, especially for dressing wounds. The numerous reports of the effectiveness of honey in wound management, including reports of several randomised controlled trials, have recently been reviewed, rapid clearance of infection from the treated wounds being a commonly recorded observation.

In almost all of these reports honey is referred to generically, there being no indication given of any awareness of the variability that generally is found in natural products. Yet the ancient physicians were aware of differences in the therapeutic value of the honeys available to them: Aristotle (384-322 BC), discussing differences in honeys, referred to pale honey being "good as a salve for sore eyes and wounds"; and Dioscorides (50 AD) stated that a pale yellow honey from Attica was the best, being "good for all rotten and hollow ulcers". Any honey can be expected to suppress infection in wounds because of its high sugar content, but dressings of sugar on a wound have to be changed more frequently than honey dressings do to maintain an osmolarity that is inhibitory to bacteria, as honey has additional antibacterial components.

Since microbiological studies have shown more than one hundred-fold differences in the potency of the antibacterial activity of various honey, best results would be expected if a honey with a high level of antibacterial activity were used in the management of infected wounds. Other therapeutic properties of honey besides its antibacterial activity are also likely to vary. An anti-inflammatory action and a stimulatory effect on angiogenesis and on the growth of granulation tissue and epithelial cells have been observed clinically and in histological studies. The components responsible for these effects have not been identified, but the anti-inflammatory action may be due to antioxidants, the level of which varies in honey. The stimulation of tissue growth may be a trophic effect, as nutrification of wounds is known to hasten the healing process: the level of the wide range of micronutrients that occur in honey also varies. Until research is carried out to ascertain the components of honey responsible for all of its therapeutic effects it will not be possible to fully standardize honey to obtain optimal effectiveness in wound management. However, where an antiseptic wound dressing is required then standardization for this effect is possible.

Several brands of honey with standardized levels of antibacterial activity are commercially available in Australia and New Zealand, but even where these are not available it is possible to assay the level of antibacterial activity of locally available honey by a simple procedure in a microbiology laboratory.

3. MATERIALS AND METHODS

3.1. GENERAL METHODS

3.1.1. Cleaning of Glassware

All the glasswares were first soaked in cleaning solution (100 g of potassium dichromate was added to 100 ml of distilled water followed by addition of 50 ml of concentrated sulphuric acid for about 12 hours and washed in tap water. Then, they were boiled soap water and washed in tap water. Finally, they were cleaned in distilled water, dried and used for the study.

3.1.2. Sterilization

All the media were sterilized in autoclaves at 15 lbs/in^2 pressure for 15 minutes. The glasswares were sterilized at 160 ^{0}C for 1 hours in Hot air oven.

3.1.3. Chemicals

The chemicals, organic solvents and reagents used in the study were of analytical reagent (AR) quality and the media were obtained from Hi-media Ltd., Mumbai.

3.2. HONEY SAMPLES SELECTED FOR PRESENT RESEARCH

  a) Kombu Honey
  b) Vembu Honey
  c) Commercially Marketed Honey - 1
  d) Commercially Marketed Honey - 2

3.3. COLLECTION OF HONEY SAMPLES

The Natural (Kombu honey and Vembu honey) and Commercial honey (Commercially marketed honey – 1 and Commercially marketed honey – 2) samples selected for the present study was collected from Alangayam, Vellore district, Tamil Nadu, India.

3.4. COLLECTION OF BACTERIAL AND FUNGAL CULTURES

Nine different bacterial cultures and One fungal yeast culture was procured from Department of Biochemistry and Microbiology, Sacred Heart College (Autonomous), Tirupattur, Tamil Nadu, India.

Gram positive bacteria

a) *Staphylococcus aureus*
b) *Bacillus cereus*
c) *Enterococcus casseliflavus.*

Gram negative bacteria

a) *Escherichia coli*
b) *Salmonella typhi*
c) *Proteus mirabilis*
d) *Klebsiella pneumonia*
e) *Shigella flexneri*
f) *Pseudomonas aeruginosa.*

Yeast

a) *Candida albicans*

3.5. CULTURE MAINTENANCE AND INOCULUM PREPARATION

3.5.1. Maintenance of test bacterial and yeast cultures

The test bacterial isolates were sub-cultures and maintained on Nutrient agar slants and the Yeast isolate *Candida albicans* were sub-cultures and maintained on Sabouraud's dextrose agar slants. The microbial slants were stored in refrigerator at 4 °C.

3.5.2. Bacterial inoculum preparation

Bacterial inoculums was prepared by inoculating a loopful of test organisms in 5 ml of Nutrient broth and incubated at 37 °C for 24 hours till a moderate turbidity was developed.

3.5.3. Yeast inoculum preparation

The inoculums of Yeast *Candida albicans* was prepared by inoculating a loopful of test organisms in 5 ml of Sabouraud's dextrose broth and incubated at room temperature for 48 hours till a moderate turbidity was developed.

3.6. DETERMINATION ANTIBACTERIAL ACTIVITY OF NATURAL AND COMMERCIAL HONEY

Mueller Hinton Agar plates were prepared and inoculated with test bacterial isolates by spreading the bacterial inoculum on the surface of the media. Wells (6 mm in diameter) were punched in the Mueller Hinton Agar. Honey samples with 75 µl/ml concentrations was mixed with 1 ml of Dimethyl sulfoxide (DMSO), mixed well and added into the well. Well containing DMSO alone act as a Negative control. The plates were incubated at 37 °C for 24 hours. The antibacterial activity was assessed by measuring the diameter of the zone of inhibition (in mm).

3.7. ANTIOXIDANT ACTIVITY BY DPPH (Diphenyl-1-picrylhydrazyl) FREE RADICAL SCAVENGING METHOD

Free radical scavenging activity of different Natural (Kombu honey and Vembu honey) and Commercial honey (Commercially marketed honey – 1 and Commercially marketed honey – 2) was measured by DPPH (Diphenyl-1-picrylhydrazyl) free radical scavenging method. A volume of 0.1 mM solution of DPPH in ethanol was prepared. Then, 1 ml of solution was added to 3 ml of different extracts in ethanol at different concentrations *viz.*, 5 µg/ml, 10 µg/ml, 15 µg/ml, 20 µg/ml, 25 µg/ml and 30 µg/ml. The Essential oil samples were solubilized with the detergent Sodium dodecyl sulphate (SDS) and their various concentrations were prepared by Dilution method. The mixture was shaken vigorously and allowed to stand at room temperature for 30 minutes. Then, absorbance was measured at 517 nm by using Spectrophotometer (UV-VIS Shimadzu). Reference standard compound being used was ascorbic acid and experiment was done in triplicate. The IC_{50} value of the sample, which is the concentration of sample required to inhibit 50 % of the DPPH free radicals was calculated using Log dose inhibition curve. Lower absorbance of the reaction mixture indicated higher free radical activity. The percent DPPH free redical scavenging effect was calculated by using following equation.

DPPH free radical Scavenging effect (%) or Percent inhibition = $A_0 - A_1/A_0 \times 100$.

Where,

A_0 = The absorbance of control reaction

A_1 = The absorbance in presence of test or standard sample

4. RESULTS AND DISCUSSION

The antimicrobial activity and antioxidant activity of the four different honey samples (two Natural honeys – Vembu honey & Kombu honey and two Commercially marketed honeys – Commercially marketed honey 1 & Commercially marketed honey 2) was studied in this present research. The antimicrobial activity of honey was studied against nine bacterial cultures (three Gram positive bacteria and six Gram negative bacteria) and one fungal yeast culture (*Candida albicans*) by Agar well diffusion method which was proposed by Kirby and Bauer. The DPPH free radicals scavenging activity of the honey samples also studied in this present research. The findings of the present research was given and discussed below.

4.1. ANTIMICROBIAL ACTIVITY OF NATURAL KOMBU HONEY

The antimicrobial activity of Natural Kombu Honey was studied against microbial pathogens and the findings were furnished in Table – 1. The Natural Kombu Honey exhibited more antimicrobial activity against bacterial pathogens and does not showed any inhibitory activity against the fungal pathogenic yeast *Candida albicans*. It was observed that the Gram negative bacteria have showed highest inhibitory activity when compared to the Gram positive bacteria. The Natural Kombu Honey showed highest inhibitory activity against the Pneumonia causing bacteria *Klebsiella pneumoniae* (35 mm in dm) followed by the Gram positive Urinary tract infection causing cocci *Staphylococcus aureus* (32 mm in dm), Typhoid causing *Salmonella typhi* (22 mm in dm), Coliform bacteria *Escherichia coli* (20 mm in dm), Urinary tract infection causing bacilli *Proteus mirabilis* (20 mm in dm) and Food borne disease causing Gram positive bacilli *Bacillus cereus* (18 mm in dm). The Natural Kombu Honey was completely resistant to *Enterococcus casseliflavus*, *Shigella flexneri*, *Pseudomonas aeruginosa* and fungal yeast *Candida albicans*. The negative control DMSO also does not showed any inhibitory activity.

Table – 1: Antimicrobial activity of Natural Kombu Honey against pathogenic microorganisms

S. No	Microorganisms	Zone of inhibition (mm in dm)	
		Natural Kombu Honey	DMSO
Gram positive bacteria			
1	*Staphylococcus aureus*	32	NZ
2	*Bacillus cereus*	18	NZ
3	*Enterococcus casseliflavus*	NZ	NZ
Gram negative bacteria			
4	*Escherichia coli*	20	NZ
5	*Salmonella typhi*	22	NZ
6	*Klebsiella pneumoniae*	35	NZ
7	*Proteus mirabilis*	20	NZ
8	*Shigella flexneri*	NZ	NZ
9	*Pseudomonas aeruginosa*	NZ	NZ
Fungi – Yeast			
10	*Candida albicans*	NZ	NZ

*NZ – No zone of inhibition

4.2. ANTIMICROBIAL ACTIVITY OF NATURAL VEMBU HONEY

The antimicrobial activity of Natural Vembu Honey was tested against microbial pathogens and the results were tabulated in Table – 2. Like Natural Kombu Honey, the Natural Vembu Honey also exhibited good antimicrobial activity against bacterial pathogens and not against the fungal pathogenic yeast *Candida albicans*. As same like Natural Kombu Honey, it was observed that the Natural Vembu Honey have showed highest inhibitory activity against Gram negative bacteria when compared to the Gram positive bacteria. The Natural Vembu Honey have showed highest zone of inhibition against the Pneumonia causing bacteria *Klebsiella pneumoniae* (38 mm in dm) followed by the Gram positive clustery arranged cocci *Staphylococcus aureus* (35 mm in dm), Typhoid causing *Salmonella typhi* (25 mm in dm) and Coliform bacteria *Escherichia coli* (20 mm in dm). The Natural Vembu Honey was completely resistant to *Bacillus subtilis, Proteus mirabilis, Enterococcus casseliflavus, Shigella flexneri, Pseudomonas aeruginosa* and fungal yeast *Candida albicans*. The negative control DMSO also does not showed any inhibitory activity.

4.3. ANTIMICROBIAL ACTIVITY OF COMMERCIALLY MARKETED HONEY - 1

The antimicrobial activity of Commercially Marketed Honey - 1 was determined against pathogenic microorganisms and the findings were given in Table – 3. Like Natural Kombu Honey and Natural Vembu Honey, the Commercially Marketed Honey - 1 also exhibited good antimicrobial activity against bacterial pathogens and not against the fungal pathogenic yeast *Candida albicans*. In contrast to the Natural Honey, it was noticed that the Commercially Marketed Honey - 1 have showed highest inhibitory activity against Gram positive bacteria when compared to the Gram negative bacteria. The Commercially Marketed Honey - 1 have showed highest zone of inhibition against the *Staphylococcus aureus* (22 mm in dm) followed by the *Klebsiella pneumoniae* (21 mm in dm), *Salmonella typhi* (12 mm in dm) and *Escherichia coli* (8 mm in dm). No zone of inhibition was recorded against *Bacillus subtilis, Proteus mirabilis, Enterococcus casseliflavus, Shigella flexneri, Pseudomonas aeruginosa* and *Candida albicans*. The negative control DMSO also does not showed any inhibitory activity.

Table – 2: Antimicrobial activity of Natural Vembu Honey against pathogenic microorganisms

S. No	Microorganisms	Zone of inhibition (mm in dm)	
		Natural Vembu Honey	**DMSO**
Gram positive bacteria			
1	*Staphylococcus aureus*	35	NZ
2	*Bacillus cereus*	NZ	NZ
3	*Enterococcus casseliflavus*	NZ	NZ
Gram negative bacteria			
4	*Escherichia coli*	22	NZ
5	*Salmonella typhi*	25	NZ
6	*Klebsiella pneumoniae*	38	NZ
7	*Proteus mirabilis*	NZ	NZ
8	*Shigella flexneri*	NZ	NZ
9	*Pseudomonas aeruginosa*	NZ	NZ
Fungi – Yeast			
10	*Candida albicans*	NZ	NZ

*NZ – No zone of inhibition

Table – 3: Antimicrobial activity of Commercially marketed Honey - 1 against pathogenic microorganisms

S. No	Microorganisms	Zone of inhibition (mm in dm)	
		Commercial Honey – 1	DMSO
Gram positive bacteria			
1	*Staphylococcus aureus*	22	NZ
2	*Bacillus cereus*	NZ	NZ
3	*Enterococcus casseliflavus*	NZ	NZ
Gram negative bacteria			
4	*Escherichia coli*	8	NZ
5	*Salmonella typhi*	12	NZ
6	*Klebsiella pneumoniae*	21	NZ
7	*Proteus mirabilis*	NZ	NZ
8	*Shigella flexneri*	NZ	NZ
9	*Pseudomonas aeruginosa*	NZ	NZ
Fungi – Yeast			
10	*Candida albicans*	NZ	NZ

*NZ – No zone of inhibition

4.4. ANTIMICROBIAL ACTIVITY OF COMMERCIALLY MARKETED HONEY - 2

The antimicrobial activity of Commercially Marketed Honey - 2 was studied against pathogenic bacteria and yeast, and the results were showed in Table - 4. Like Natural Kombu Honey, Natural Vembu Honey and Commercially Marketed Honey – 1, the Commercially Marketed Honey - 2 also exhibited an increased antimicrobial activity against bacterial pathogens and not against the fungal pathogenic yeast *Candida albicans*. The antimicrobial activity of the Commercially Marketed Honey – 2 is more when compared to Commercially Marketed Honey – 1. In contrast to the Commercially Marketed Honey - 1 and similar to Natural Honey, it was recorded that the Commercially Marketed Honey - 2 have showed highest inhibitory activity against Gram negative bacteria when compared to the Gram positive bacteria. The Commercially Marketed Honey - 1 have showed highest zone of inhibition against the *Klebsiella pneumoniae* (25 mm in dm) followed by the *Staphylococcus aureus* (23 mm in dm), *Salmonella typhi* (15 mm in dm) and *Escherichia coli* (14 mm in dm). No zone of inhibition was recorded against *Bacillus subtilis*, *Proteus mirabilis*, *Enterococcus casseliflavus*, *Shigella flexneri*, *Pseudomonas aeruginosa* and *Candida albicans*. The negative control DMSO also does not showed any inhibitory activity.

4.5. ANTIOXIDANT ACTIVITY OF NATURAL AND COMMERCIAL HONEY BY DPPH (Diphenyl-1-picrylhydrazyl) FREE RADICAL SCAVENGING METHOD

The Antioxidant activity of the Natural honey and Commercial honey was studied by DPPH (Diphenyl-1-picrylhydrazyl) free radical scavenging activity and the results were presented in Table – 5. It was clear that the Natural Vembu Honey (85 %) was having more DPPH free radical scavenging activity followed by Natural Kombu Honey (75 %), Commercially marketed honey – 1 (60 %) and Commercially marketed honey – 2 (42 %). It was found that the Natural honey is having highest Antioxidant activity than the Commercial honey.

Table – 4: Antimicrobial activity of Commercially marketed Honey - 2 against pathogenic microorganisms

S. No	Microorganisms	Zone of inhibition (mm in dm)	
		Commercial Honey – 1	DMSO
Gram positive bacteria			
1	*Staphylococcus aureus*	23	NZ
2	*Bacillus cereus*	NZ	NZ
3	*Enterococcus casseliflavus*	NZ	NZ
Gram negative bacteria			
4	*Escherichia coli*	14	NZ
5	*Salmonella typhi*	15	NZ
6	*Klebsiella pneumoniae*	25	NZ
7	*Proteus mirabilis*	NZ	NZ
8	*Shigella flexneri*	NZ	NZ
9	*Pseudomonas aeruginosa*	NZ	NZ
Fungi – Yeast			
10	*Candida albicans*	NZ	NZ

*NZ – No zone of inhibition

Table – 5: DPPH free radical scavenging activity of different Natural and Commercial Honey

S. No	Essential Oils	Optical Density (at 520 nm)	DPPH free radical Scavenging effect (%)
1	Natural Kombu Honey	0.25	75
2	Natural Vembu Honey	0.15	85
3	Commercially Marketed Honey - 1	0.40	60
4	Commercially Marketed Honey - 2	0.58	42

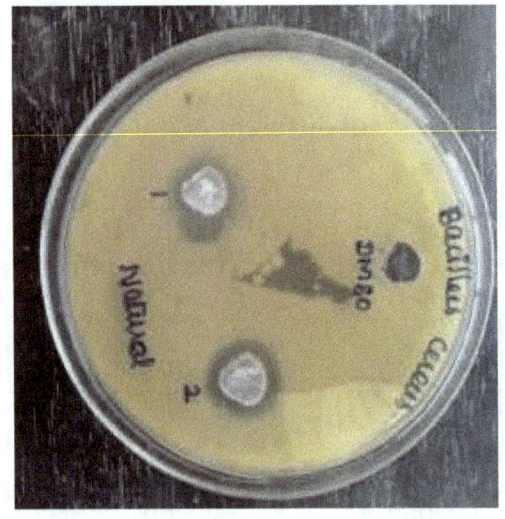
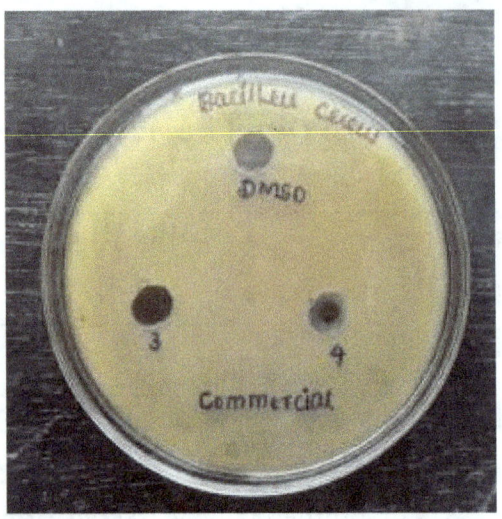

1 – Kombu honey, 2 – Vembu honey, 3 – Commercially marketed honey 1 and 4 - – Commercially marketed honey 1

Figure – 1: Antibacterial activity of Natural and Commercial honey against *Bacillus cereus*

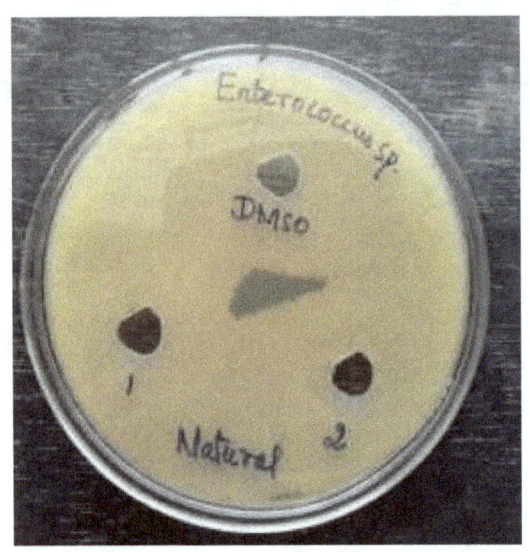
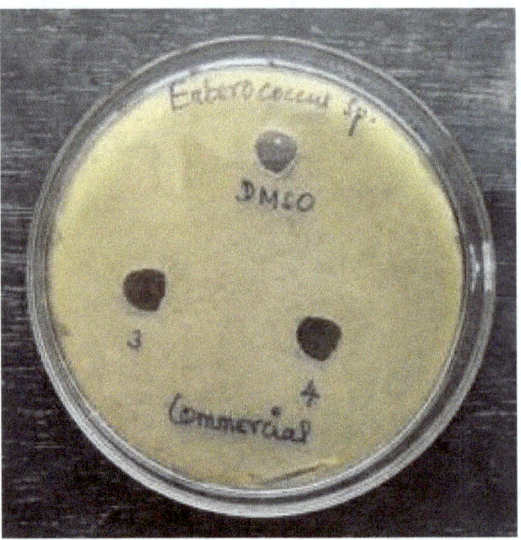

1 – Kombu honey, 2 – Vembu honey, 3 – Commercially marketed honey 1 and 4 - – Commercially marketed honey 1

Figure – 2: Antibacterial activity of Natural and Commercial honey against *Enterococcus casseliflavus*

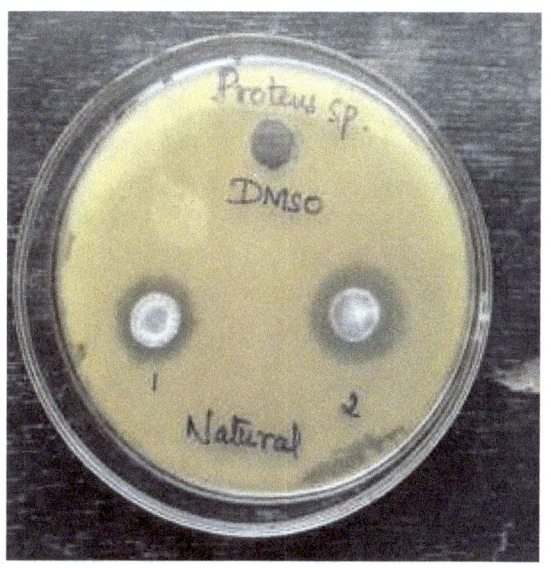 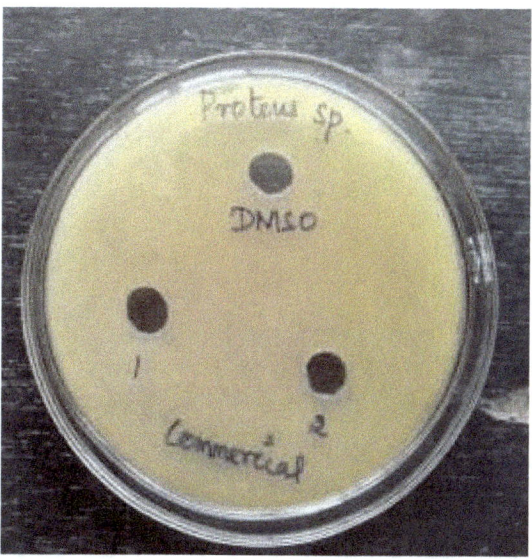

1 – Kombu honey, 2 – Vembu honey, 3 – Commercially marketed honey 1 and 4 - – Commercially marketed honey 1

Figure – 3: Antibacterial activity of Natural and Commercial honey against *Proteus mirabilis*

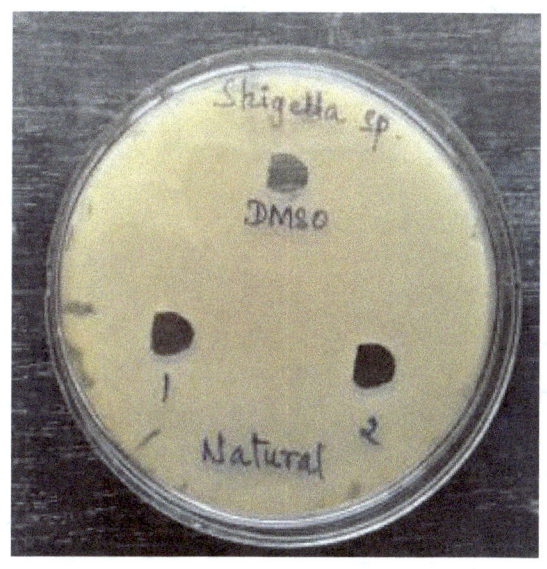 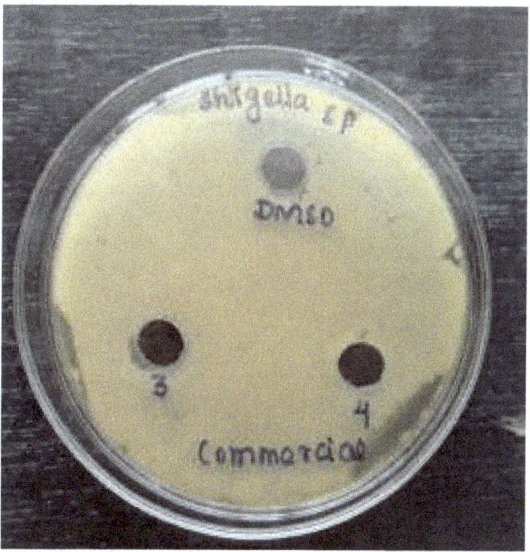

1 – Kombu honey, 2 – Vembu honey, 3 – Commercially marketed honey 1 and 4 - – Commercially marketed honey 1

Figure – 4: Antibacterial activity of Natural and Commercial honey against *Shigella flexneri*

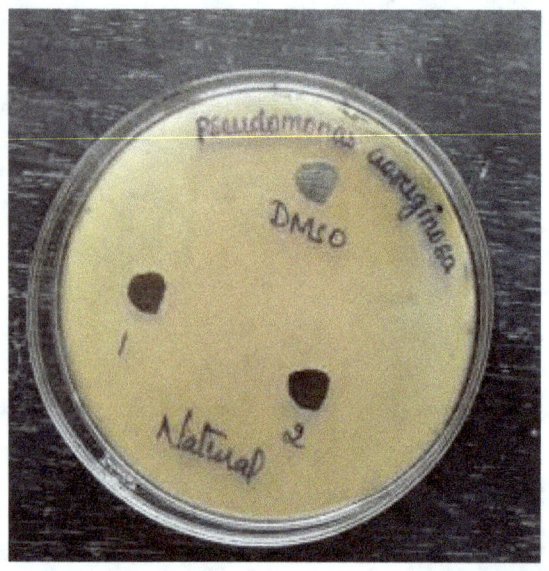 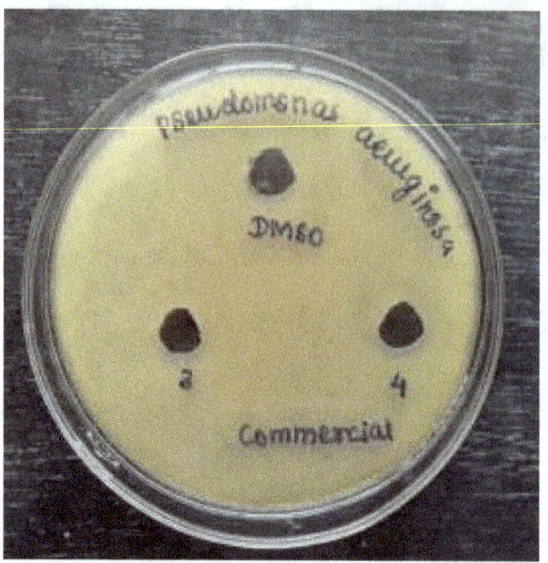

1 – Kombu honey, 2 – Vembu honey, 3 – Commercially marketed honey 1 and
4 - Commercially marketed honey 2

Figure – 5: Antibacterial activity of Natural and Commercial honey against
Pseudomonas aeruginosa

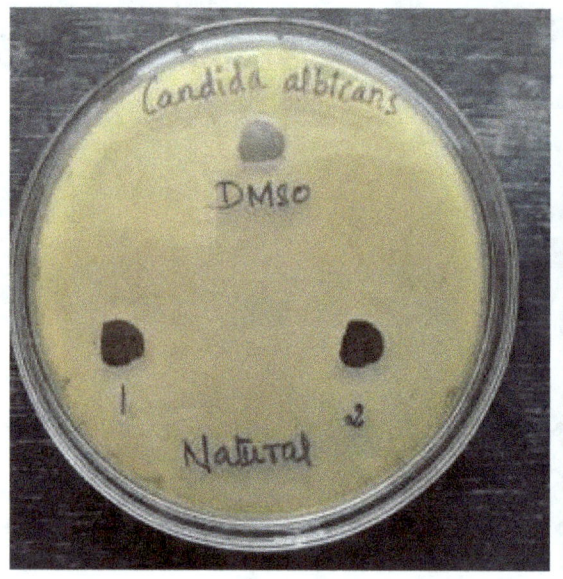 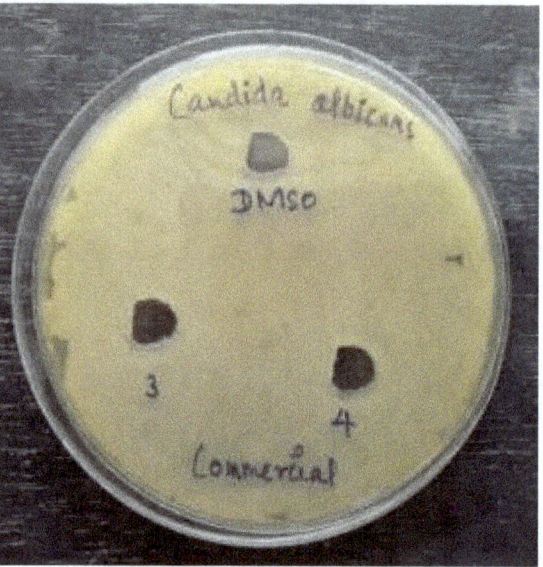

1 – Kombu honey, 2 – Vembu honey, 3 – Commercially marketed honey 1 and
4 - Commercially marketed honey 2

Figure – 6: Anticandidal activity of Natural and Commercial honey against
Candida albicans

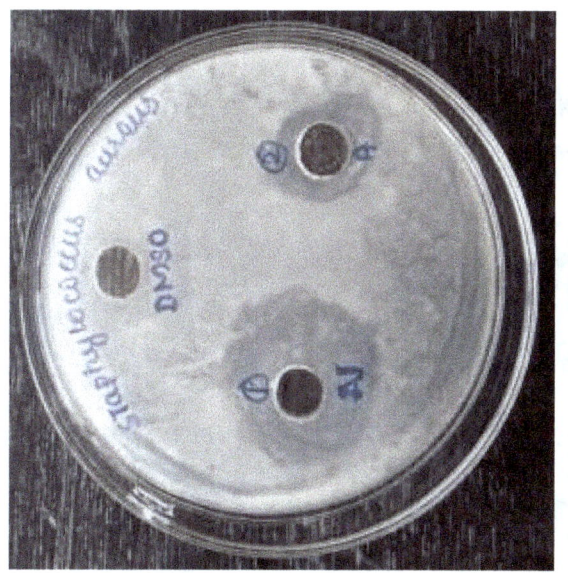
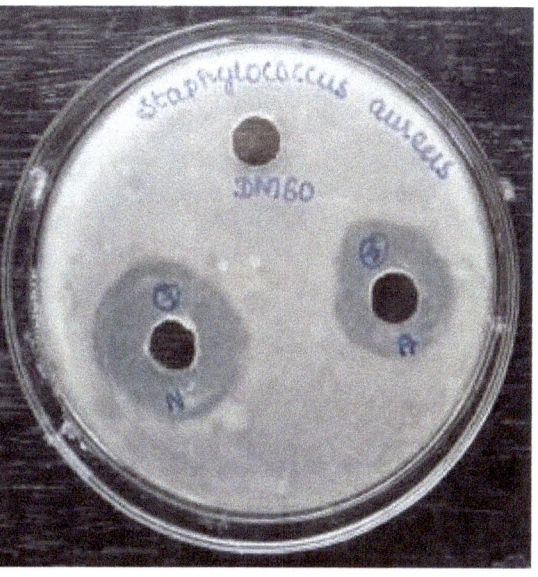

1 – Kombu honey, 2 – Commercially marketed honey 1, 3 – Vembu honey and
4 - Commercially marketed honey 2

Figure – 7: Antibacterial activity of Natural and Commercial honey against
Staphylococcus aureus

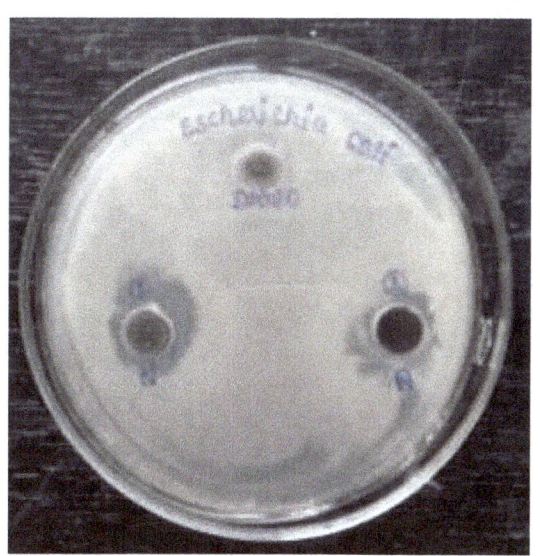
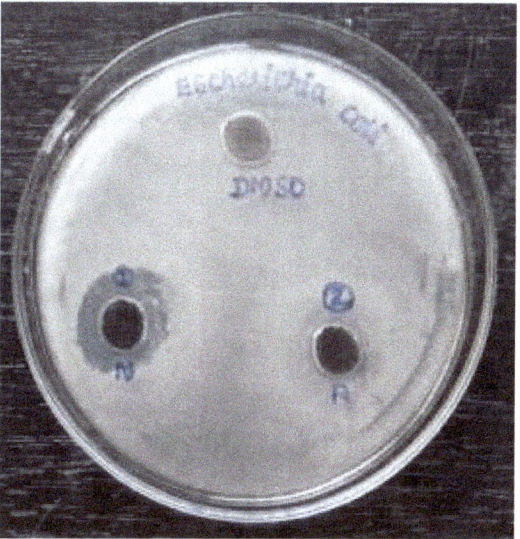

1 – Kombu honey, 2 – Commercially marketed honey 1, 3 – Vembu honey and
4 - Commercially marketed honey 2

Figure – 8: Antibacterial activity of Natural and Commercial honey against
Escherichia coli

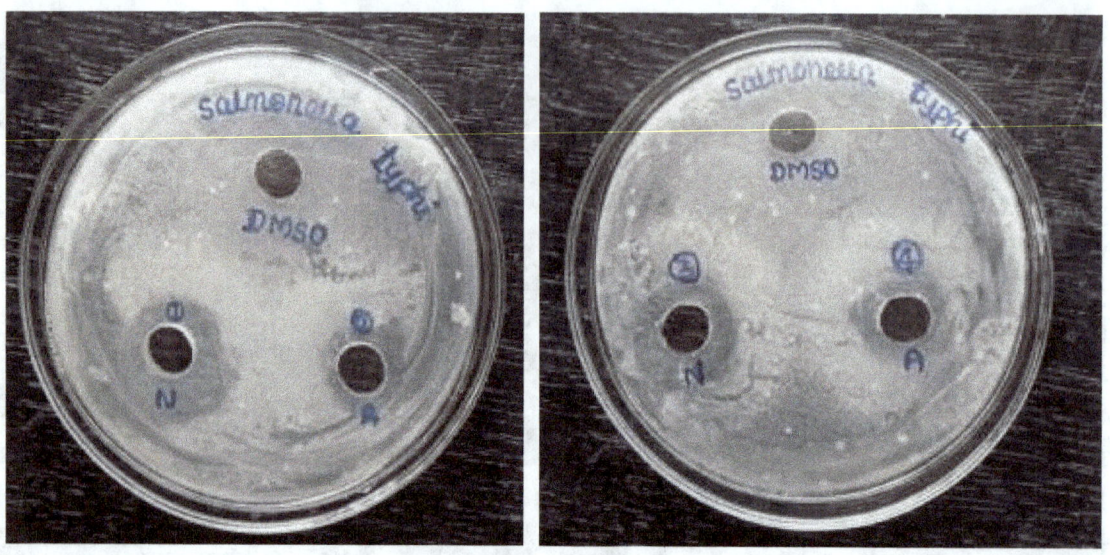

1 – Kombu honey, 2 – Commercially marketed honey 1, 3 – Vembu honey and
4 - Commercially marketed honey 2

Figure – 9: Antibacterial activity of Natural and Commercial honey against
Salmonella typhi

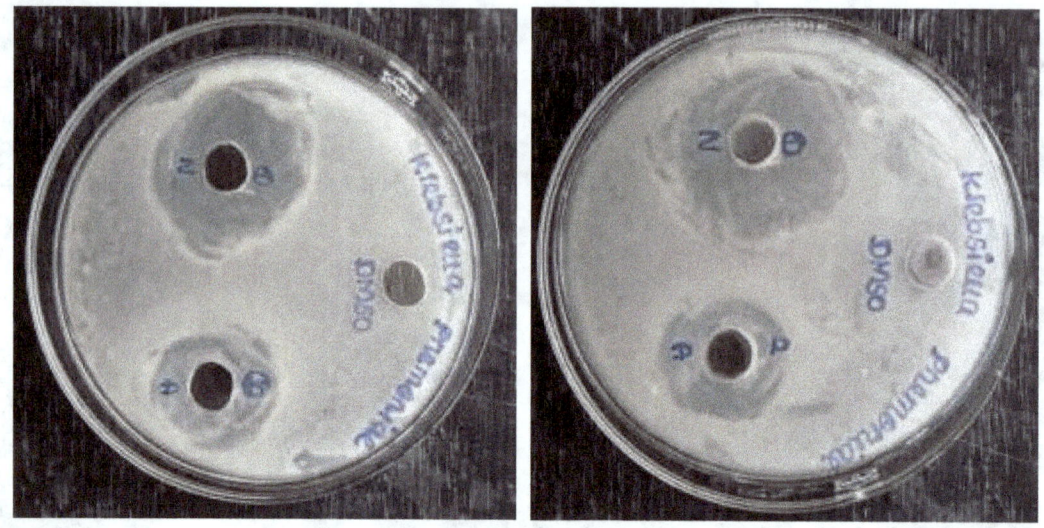

1 – Kombu honey, 2 – Commercially marketed honey 1, 3 – Vembu honey and
4 - Commercially marketed honey 2

Figure – 10: Antibacterial activity of Natural and Commercial honey against
Klebsiella pneumoniae

The pharmacological activity of honey was studied by various researchers in various microorganisms like bacteria and fungi. Broadly, in our study we found that the Natural honey was the good for the treatment of bacterial diseases than the Commercial honey. The same was also observed in the case of Antioxidant activity. Both the natural honey and commercial honey has not showed any inhibitory activity against *Candida albicans*. The Natural honey samples have showed best Antioxidant activity when compared to the Commercially marketed honey. Both the Natural Kombu Honey and Natural Vembu Honey have showed more or less similar activity against pathogenic microorganisms. The Natural Kombu Honey has showed Broad spectrum activity against pathogenic bacteria by providing inhibitory activity against many tested bacterial isolates. The Natural Vembu Honey has showed Narrow spectrum activity against pathogenic bacteria by providing inhibitory activity against limited tested bacterial isolates. The Natural Kombu Honey has showed less inhibitory activity against many bacterial isolates but in contrast, the Natural Vembu Honey more inhibitory activity against selected bacterial isolates.

Honey is the only food material which cannot be spoiled for hundreds of years and does not allow its container also to spoil. But, the commercial honeys are available in marked with expiry date. This one character is enough to propose the natural honey as the best one in all the ways than the Commercial honey.

Sampath Kumar (2010) revealed the activity of Honey samples against wound infections and its management. Srisayam and Chantawannakul (2010) investigated the antifungal activity of honey samples against two fungal yeast isolates *viz.*, *Candida albicans* and *Saccharomyces cerevisiae*. They showed that the honey samples are completely resistant to *Candida albicans* and *Saccharomyces cerevisiae*. The finding of the research of Srisayam and Chantawannakul (2010) was similar with the results of our present study. In our present study, we studied the antimicrobial activity of Natural and Commercial honey samples against the fungal yeast *Candida albicans*. We also found that the *Candida albicans* was totally resistance to both Natural and Commercial honey samples. According to the studies of Kirnpal Kaur *et al.* (2011), it was found that Tualang honey had an important role in bactericidal effects and bacteriostatic effects in the treatment of burns and several wounds by using dressings soaked with this honey.

Recently, Kalidasan *et al.* (2017) investigated the antibacterial activity of two Malan honey, Kombu honey and two Commercial honeys. They found that the Natural honey has showed more antibacterial activity than the Commercial honey. The finding of the present research was similar with the results of Kalidasan *et al.* (2017). They also concluded that the Natural honey was the best source for treating bacterial infection than the Commercial honey.

5. CONCLUSION

Natural honey showed maximum Antimicrobial activity and Antioxidant activity than Commercially marketed honey. It was showed that the honey samples does not exhibited antimicrobial activity against the yeast *Candida albicans*. The pharmacological activity of Vembu honey was comparatively high when compared to the Kombu honey. All the honey samples are resistant to *Candida albicans*, *Shigella flexneri*, *Enterococcus casseliflavus* and *Pseudomonas aeruginosa*. Highest inhibitory activity was observed against *Klebsiella pneumoniae* and *Staphylococcus aureus*. In conclusion, honey is effective against the bacterial pathogens which are frequently causing Urinary tract infection and Neonatal sepsis, and it is the "SWEET MEDICINE" for bacterial infections. We also recommend the Women and Infants to take the Vembu honey regularly for preventing them from the Urinary tract infection and Neonatal sepsis.

6. REFERENCES

1) Adams, C. J., Manley Harris, M and Molan, P. C. 2009. The origin of methylglyoxal in New Zealand manuka (*Leptospermum scoparium*) honey. *Carbohydrate Research,* 344: 1050 - 1053.

2) Alves Da Silva, R., Arraes Maia, G., Machado De Souza, P H. and Correia Da Costa, J. M. 2006. Composição e propriedades terapêuticas do mel de abelha. *Alimentos Nutrição,* 17 (1): 113 - 120.

3) Al-Waili, N. S. 2004. Natural honey lowers plasma glucose, C-reactive protein, homocysteine, and blood lipids in healthy, diabetic, and hyperlipidemic subjects: Comparison with dextrose and sucrose. *Journal of Medicine and Food,* 7: 100 – 107.

4) Al-Waili, N. S. 2003. Topical application of natural honey, beeswax and olive oil mixture for atopic dermatitis or psoriasis: partially controlled, single - blinded study. *Complementary Therapies in Medicine*, 11(4): 226 – 234.

5) Anklam, E. 1998. A review of the analytical methods to determine the geographical and botanical origin of honey. *Food Chemistry*, 63 (4): 549 - 562.

6) Aronne, G and Micco, D. E. 2010. Traditional melissopalynology integrated by multivariate analysis and sampling methods to improve botanical and geographical characterization of honeys. *Plant Biosynthesis,* 144: 833 - 840.

7) Assia, A and Ali, L. 2015. Enzymes activities, hydroxymethylfurfural content and pollen spectrum of some Algerian honey. *African Journal of Agricultural Research,* 10: 613 - 622.

8) Aysan, E., Ayar, E., Aren, A and Cifter, C. 2002. The role of intraperitoneal honey administration in preventing postoperative peritoneal adhesions. *European Journal of Gynecology and Reproduction Biology,* 104(2): 152 – 155.

9) Bang L. M., Buntting C and Molan P. 2003. Peroxide production in honey and its implications. *Journal of Alternative and Complement Medicine*, 9: 267 - 273.

10) Baroni, M. V., Nores, M. L., Diaz Mdel, P., Chiabrando, G. A., Fassano, J. P., Costa, C and Wunderlin, D. A. 2006. Determination of volatile organic compound patterns characteristic of five unifloral honey by solid-phase microextraction-gas chromatography-mass spectrometry coupled to chemometrics. *Journal of Agricultural and Food Chemistry,* 54: 7235 - 7241.

11) Beck, B. F and Smedley D. 1997. Honey and your health. New York, McBride Publishing (originally published in 1944).

12) Bauer, A. W., Kirby, W. M. M., Sherris, J. C and Turck, M. 1966. Antibiotic susceptibility testing by a standardized single disk method. *American Journal of Clinical Pathology*, 45 (4): 493 - 496.

13) Bertrams, J., Kunz, N., Müller, M., Kammerer, D and Stintzing, F. C. 2013. Phenolic compounds as marker compounds for botanical origin determination of German propolis samples based on TLC and TLC-MS. *Journal of Applied Botany and Food Quality,* 86: 143 – 153.

14) Beutler, J. A. 2009. Natural products as a foundation for drug discovery. *Current Protocols in Pharmacology*, 46: 115 - 122.

15) Blair, S. E., Cokcetin, N. N., Harry, E. J and Carter, D. A. 2009. The unusual antibacterial activity of medical-grade *Leptospermum* honey: antibacterial spectrum, resistance and transcriptome analysis. *European Journal of Clinical Microbiology and Infectious Diseases,* 28: 1199 – 1208.

16) Bobis, O., Marghitas, L., Rindt, I. K., Niculae, M and Dezmirean, D. 2008. Honeydew honey: correlations between Chemical composition, antioxidant capacity and Antibacterial effect. *Lucrări stiinŃifice Zootehnie si Biotehnologii*, 41(2): 271- 2 77.

17) Bogdanov, S. 2006. Contaminants of bee products. *Apidologie*, 38: 1 - 18.

18) Bogdanov, S., Martin P and Lüllman, C. 1997. Harmonised methods of the European Honey Comission. *Apidologie,* 3: 1 - 59.

19) Bogdanov, S., Ruoff, K and Oddo, L. P. 2004. Physico-chemical methods for the characterization of unifloral honeys: a review. *Apidologie*, 35: S4 - S17.

20) Brady, N., Molan, P and Bang, L. 2004. A survey of non-manuka New Zealand honeys for antibacterial and antifungal activities. *Journal of Apiculture Research*, 43: 47 – 52.

21) Brudzynski, K and Kim, L. 2011. Storage induced chemical changes in active components of honey deregulate its antibacterial activity. *Food Chemistry*, 126: 1155 - 1163.

22) Brudzynski, K and Lannigan, R. 2012. Mechanism of honey bacteriostatic action against MRSA and VRE involves hydroxyl radicals generated from honey's hydrogen peroxide. *Frontiers in microbiology*, 3: 36 - 40.

23) Brudzynski, K., Abubaker, K and Miotto, D. 2012. Unraveling a mechanism of honey antibacterial action: Polyphenol or H_2O_2 - induced oxidative effect on bacterial cell growth and on DNA degradation. *Food Chemistry*, 133: 329 - 336.

24) Brudzynski, K., Abubaker, K., Laurent, M and Castle, A. 2011. Re-examining the role of hydrogen peroxide in bacteriostatic and bactericidal activities of honey. *Frontiers in microbiology*, 2: 213.

25) Bruggink, A., Roos, E. C and De Vroom, E. 1998. Penicillin acylase in the industrial production of β-lactam antibiotics. *Organic Process Research and Development*, 2: 128 - 133.

26) Bruni, I., Galimberti, A., Caridi, L., Scaccabarozzi, D., De Mattia, F., Casiraghi, M and Labra, M. 2015. A DNA barcoding approach to identify plant species in multiflower honey. *Food Chemistry*, 170: 308 - 315.

27) Bucekova, M., Valachova, I., Kohutova, L., Prochazka, E., Klaudiny, J and Majtan, J. 2014. Honeybee glucose oxidase - its expression in honeybee workers and comparative analyses of its content and H_2O_2 - mediated antibacterial activity in natural honeys. *Nature* 101: 661 - 670.

28) Butler, M. S., Robertson, A. B and Cooper, M. A. 2014. Natural product and natural product derived drugs in clinical trials. *Natural Product Reports,* 31, 1612 - 1661.

29) Cai, Y., Luo, Q., Sun, M and Corke, H. 2004. Antioxidant activity and phenolic compounds of 112 traditional Chinese medicinal plants associated with anticancer. *Life Sciences,* 74: 2157 - 2184.

30) Casteels, P., Ampe, C., Jacobs, F and Tempst, P. 1993. Functional and chemical characterization of Hymenoptaecin, an antibacterial polypeptide that is infection-inducible in the honeybee (*Apis mellifera*). *Journal of Biological Chemistry,* 268: 7044 - 7054.

31) Castro-Vazquez, L., Diaz - Maroto, M. C., González - Viñas, M. A., De La Fuente, E and Pérez - Coello, M. S. 2008. Influence of storage conditions on chemical composition and sensory properties of citrus honey. *Journal of Agricultural and Food Chemistry,* 56: 1999 - 2006.

32) Conti, M. E. 2000. Lazio region (Central Italy) honeys: a survey of mineral content and typical quality parameters. *Food Control,* 11: 459 – 463.

33) Cooper, R. A., Halas, E and Molan, P. C. 2002. The efficacy of honey in inhibiting strains of *Pseudomonas aeruginosa* from infected burns. *The Journal of Burn Care and Rehabilitation,* 23: 366 - 370.

34) Cooper, R. A., Molan, P. C and Harding, K. G. 2002. The sensitivity to honey of Gram positive cocci of clinical significance isolated from wounds. *Journal of Applied Microbiology,* 93: 857 – 863.

35) Cortes, M. E., Vigil, P and Montenegro, G. 2011. The medicinal value of honey: a review on its benefits to human health, with a special focus on its effects on glycemic regulation. *Bioresource Technology,* 38(2): 303 - 317.

36) Cragg, G. M and Newman, D. J. 2013. Natural products: a continuing source of novel drug leads. *Biochimica et Biophysica Acta,* 1830: 3670 - 3695.

37) Crane, E and Visscher, P. K. 2009. Chapter 121 - Honey, In: Vincent H. Resh and Ring T. Carde, Editor(s), Encyclopedia of Insects (Second Edition), Academic Press, San Diego, Pages 459-461.

38) Crane, E. 1975. Honey - A comprehensive survey. First Heinemann London.
39) Crane, E. 1999. The World History of Beekeeping and Honey Hunting. Gerald Duckworth and Co. Ltd, London.
40) Cuevas Glory, L. F., Pino, J. A., Santiago, L. S and Sauri-Duch, E. 2007. A review of volatile analytical methods for determining the botanical origin of honey. *Food Chemistry,* 103: 1032 - 1043.
41) David, B., Wolfender, J. L and Dias, D. 2014. The pharmaceutical industry and natural products: historical status and new trends. *Phytochemistry Reviews*, 36: 1 - 17.
42) Davidson, B. S. 1995. New dimensions in natural products research: cultured marine microorganisms. *Current Opinion in Biotechnology,* 6: 284 - 291.
43) Derek, D., Schramm, D., Malina Karim, T., Heather R. Schrader, Roberta R. Holt, Marcia Cardetti and Carl L. Keen. 2013. *Journal of Agriculture and Food Chemistry*, 51(6): 1732 – 1735.
44) Deurenberg, R. H and Stobberingh, E. E. 2008. The evolution of Staphylococcus aureus. *Infection, Genetics and Evolution,* 8: 747 - 763.
45) Dixon, R. A and Pasinetti, G. M. 2010. Flavonoids and isoflavonoids: from plant biology to agriculture and neuroscience. *Plant Physiology,* 154: 453 - 457.
46) Dong, R., Zheng, Y and Xu, B. 2013. Phenolic profiles and antioxidant capacities of chinese unifloral honeys from different botanical and geographical sources. *Food and Bioprocess Technology,* 6: 762 - 770.
47) Dossey, A. T. 2010. Insects and their chemical weaponry: New potential for drug discovery. *Natural Product Reports,* 27: 1737 - 1757.
48) Eldridge, G. R., Vervoort, H. C., Lee, C. M., Cremin, P. A., Williams, C. T., Hart, S. M., Goering, M. G., O'neil - Johnso, M and Zeng, L. 2002. High - Throughput Method for the Production and Analysis of Large Natural Product Libraries for Drug Discovery. *Analytical Chemistry,* 74: 3963 - 3971.
49) Erlanson, D. 2012. Introduction to fragment-based drug discovery. *In:* DAVIES, T. G. & HYVÖNEN, M. (eds.) *Fragment-Based Drug Discovery and X-Ray Crystallography.* Springer Berlin Heidelberg.

50) Escuredo, O., Silva, L. R., Valentão, P., Seijo, M. C and Andrade, P. B. 2012. Assessing *Rubus* honey value: Pollen and phenolic compounds content and antibacterial capacity. *Food Chemistry,* 130: 671 - 678.

51) Fleming, A. 1929. On the antibacterial action of cultures of a *penicillium*, with special reference to their use in the isolation of *B. influenzae*. *International Journal of Experimental Pathology,* 10: 226 - 236.

52) Fontana, R., Mendes, M. A., Souza, B. M. D., Konno, K., Cesar, L. L. M. M., Malaspina, O and Palma, M. S. 2004. Jelleines: a family of antimicrobial peptides from the Royal Jelly of honeybees (*Apis mellifera*). *Peptides,* 25: 919 - 928.

53) Free, J. B. 1982. Bees and mankind. Boston: George Allen and Unwin.

54) Galimberti, A., De Mattia, F., Bruni, I., Scaccabarozzi, D., Sandionigi, A., Barbuto, M., Casiraghi, M and Labra, M. 2014. A DNA barcoding approach to characterize pollen collected by honeybees. *PLoS ONE,* 9: e109363.

55) Gheldof, N and Engeseth, N. J. 2002. Antioxidant capacity of honeys from various floral sources based on the determination of oxygen radical absorbance capacity and inhibition of in vitro lipoprotein oxidation in human serum samples. *Journal of Agriculture and Food Chemistry*, 50: 3050 – 3055.

56) Golob, T., Dobersek, U., Kump, P and Necemer, M. 2005. Determination of trace and minor elements in Slovenian honey by total reflection X-ray fluorescence spectroscopy. *Food Chemistry,* 91: 593 – 600.

57) Haffejee, I. E and Moosa, A. 1985. Honey in the treatment of infantile gastroenteritis. *Brazil Medical Journal,* 290: 1866 - 1867.

58) Harvey, A. 2000. Strategies for discovering drugs from previously unexplored natural products. *Drug Discovery Today,* 5: 294 - 300.

59) Harvey, A. L., Edrada Ebel, R and Quinn, R. J. 2015. The re-emergence of natural products for drug discovery in the genomics era. *Nature Reviews Drug Discovery,* 14: 111 - 129.

60) Havenhand, G. 2010. London, UK, Kyle Cathie Limited.

61) Henriques, A. F. F. M. 2006. The antibacterial activity of honey. PhD Thesis. University of Wales Institute Cardiff.

62) Henriques, A. F., Jenkins, R. E., Burton, N.F and Cooper, R. A. 2010. The intracellular effects of manuka honey on *Staphylococcus aureus*. *European Journal of Clinical Microbiology and Infectious Disease*, 29(1): 45 - 50.

63) Hopkins, B. J., Hodgson, W. C and Sutherland, S. K. 1994. Pharmacological studies of stonefish (*Synanceja trachynis*) venom. *Toxicon*, 32: 1197 - 1210.

64) Ilyasov, R., Gaifullina, L., Saltykova, E., Poskryakov, A and Nikolenko, A. 2012. Review of the expression of antimicrobial peptide defensin in honey bees *Apis Mellifera* L. *Journal of Apicultural Science*, 56: 115.

65) Irish, J., Blair, S and Carter, D. A. 2011. The antibacterial activity of honey derived from Australian flora. *PLoS ONE*, 6: e18229.

66) Isla, M. I., Craig, A., Ordonz, R., Zampini, C., Sayago, J., Bedascarrasbure, E., Alvarez, A., Salomón, V and Maldonado, L. 2011. Physico chemical and bioactive properties of honeys from Northwestern Argentina. *LWT - Food Science and Technology*, 44: 1922 - 1930.

67) Jerkovic, I., Marijanovic, Z and Staver, M. M. 2011. Screening of natural organic volatiles from prunus mahalebl. Honey: Coumarin and vomifoliol as nonspecific biomarkers. *Molecules*, 16: 2507 - 2518.

68) Jerkovic, I., Mastelic, J and Marijanovic, Z. 2006. A variety of volatile compounds as markers in unifloral honey from dalmatian sage (*Salvia officinalis* L.). *Chemistry and Biodiversity*, 3: 1307 - 1316.

69) Jones, R. 2009. Honey and healing through the ages. *Journal of Api Product and Api Medical Science* 1(1): 2 - 5.

70) Kalidasan, G., Saranraj, P., Ragul, V and Sivasakthi, S. 2017. Antibacterial activity of Natural and Commercial Honey – A comparative study. *Advances in Biological Research*, 11(6): 365 – 372.

71) Kalogeropoulos, N., Konteles, S. J., Troullidou, E., Mourtzinos, I and Karathanos, V. T. 2009. Chemical composition, antioxidant activity and antimicrobial properties of propolis extracts from Greece and Cyprus. *Food Chemistry,* 116, 452 - 461.

72) Kandil, A., El - Banby, M., Abdel - Wahed, G. K., Abdel - Gawwad, M., Fayez, M. 1987. Curative properties of true floral and false non-floral honeys on induced gastric ulcers. *Journal of Drug Research,* 17: 103 – 106.

73) Kaskoniene, V and Venskutonis, P. R. 2010. Floral markers in honey of various botanical and geographic origins: A review. *Comprehensive Reviews in Food Science and Food Safety,* 9: 620 - 634.

74) Katarina, B., Klaudiny, J., Kopernicky, J and Simuth, J. 2002. Identification of honeybee peptide active against *Paenibacillus larvae* larvae through bacterial growth-inhibition assay on polyacrylamide gel. *Apidologie,* 33: 259 - 269.

75) Kirnpal Kaur, B. S., Tan, H. T., Boukraa, L. and Gan, S. H. 2011. Different solid phase extraction fractions of Tualang (*Koompassia excelsa*) honey demonstrated diverse antibacterial properties against wound and enteric bacteria. *Journal of Apiproduct and Apimedical Science,* 3 (1): 59 - 65.

76) Klaudiny, J., Albert, S., Bachanova, K., Kopernicky, J and Simuth, J. 2005. Two structurally different defensin genes, one of them encoding a novel defensin isoform, are expressed in honeybee *Apis mellifera*. *Insect Biochemistry and Molecular Biology,* 35: 11 - 22.

77) Kubota, M., Tsuji, M., Nishimoto, M., Wongchawalit, J., Okuyama, M., Mori, H., Matsui, H., Surarit, R., Svasti, J., Kimura, A and Chiba, S. 2004. Localization of α-glucosidases I, II, and III in organs of European honeybees, *Apis mellifera* L., and the origin of α-glucosidase in honey. *Bioscience, Biotechnology, and Biochemistry,* 68: 2346 - 2352.

78) Kwakman, P. H. S and Zaat, S. A. J. 2012. Antibacterial components of honey. *IUBMB Life,* 64, 48-55.

79) Kwakman, P. H., Te Velde, A. A., De Boer, L., Speijer, D., Vandenbroucke-Grauls, C. M and Zaat, S. A. 2010. How honey kills bacteria. *FASEB Journal,* 24: 2576 - 2582.

80) Laid Boukraa. 2008. Synergistic action of starch and honey against *Candida albicans* in correlation with diastase number. *Brazilian Journal of Microbiology,* 39: 40 - 43.

81) Levy, S. B and Marshall, B. 2004. Antibacterial resistance worldwide: causes, challenges and responses. *Nature Medicine,* 10: S122 – S129.

82) Lin, L. Z and Harnly, J. M. 2007. A screening method for the identification of glycosylated flavonoids and other phenolic compounds using a standard analytical approach for all plant materials. *Journal of Agricultural and Food Chemistry,* 55: 1084 - 1096.

83) Lotfy, M., Badra, G., Burham, W and Alenzi, F. Q. 2006. Combined use of honey, bee propolis and myrrh in healing a deep, infected wound in a patient with diabetes mellitus. *Brazilian Journal of Biomedical Science,* 63: 171 - 173.

84) Manyi Loh, C. E., Clarke, A. M and Ndip, R. N. 2012. Detection of phytoconstituents in column fractions of n-hexane extract of gold crest honey exhibiting Anti-*Helicobacter pylori* activity. *Archives of Medical Research,* 43: 197 - 204.

85) Manyi Loh, C. E., Clarke, A. M., Green, E and Ndip, R. N. 2013. Inhibitory and bactericidal activity of selected South African honeys and their solvent extracts against *Helicobacter pylori*. *Pakistan Journal of Pharmaceutical Sciences,* 26: 897 - 906.

86) Manyi Loh, C. E., Ndip, R. N and Clarke, A. M. 2011. Volatile compounds in honey: A review on their involvement in aroma, botanical origin determination and potential biomedical activities. *International Journal of Molecular Sciences,* 12: 9514 - 9532.

87) Manyi Loh, C. E., Clarke, A. M and Ndip, R. N. 2011. An overview of honey: Therapeutic properties and contribution in nutrition and human health. *African Journal of Microbiology Research,* 5(8): 844 - 852.

88) Mateo, R and Bosch Reig F. 1998. Classification of Spanish Unifloral Honeys by Discriminant Analysis of Electrical Conductivity, Color, Water Content, Sugars, and pH. *Journal of Agriculture and Food Chemistry*, 46: 393 - 400.

89) Mathews, K. A and Binnington A. G. 2002. Wound management using honey. *Journal of Veterinary Science and Technology,* 24: 53 - 60.

90) Mato, I., Huidobro, J. F., Simal Lozano, J and Sancho, M. T. 2003. Significance of non aromatic organic acids in honey. *Journal of Food Protection,* 66(12): 2371 - 2376.

91) Matsunaga, S., Fusetani, N and Konosu, S. 1985. Bioactive marine metabolites VII. Structures of discodermins B, C, and D, antimicrobial peptides from the marine sponge discodermia kiiensis. *Tetrahedron Letters,* 26: 855 - 856.

92) Mavric, E., Wittmann, S and Henle, T. 2008. Identification and quantification of methyl glyoxal as the dominant antibacterial constituent of manuka (*Leptospermum scoparium*) honeys from New Zealand. *Molecular Nutrition and Food Research*, 52: 483 - 489.

93) Melliou, E and Chinou, I. 2011. Chemical constituents of selected unifloral Greek bee-honeys with antimicrobial activity. *Food Chemistry,* 129: 284 - 290.

94) Miki Fukuda. 2011. Jungle Honey Enhances Immune Function and Antitumor Activity, Hindawi Publishing Corporation, Evidence-Based Complementary and Alternative Medicin, Article ID 908743, 8.

95) Mohapatra, D. P., Thakur, V and Brar, S. K. 2011. Antibacterial efficacy of raw and processed honey. *Biotechnology Research International,* 20: 1 - 6.

96) Molan, P. C. 2001. Why honey is effective as a medicine. 2. The scientific explanation of its effects. *Bee World,* 82(1): 22 - 40.

97) Molan, P. C. 2006. The evidence supporting the use of honey as a wound dressing. *International Journal of Low Extreme Wounds*, 5: 40 - 54.

98) Molan P. C and Allen, K. L. 1996. The effect of gamma-irradiation on the antibacterial activity of honey. *Journal of Pharmacogeny and Pharmacology,* 48 (11): 1206 - 1209.

99) Molan, P. C. 1992. The antibacterial activity of honey. *Bee World,* 73: 5 – 28.

100) Molan, P. C. 2006. Using honey in wound care. *International Journal of Clinical Aromatherapy,* 3(2): 21 - 24.

101) Morais, M., Moreira, L., Feas, X and Estevinho, L. M. 2011. Honey bee - collected pollen from five Portuguese Natural Parks: Palynological origin, phenolic content, antioxidant properties and antimicrobial activity. *Food and Chemical Toxicology,* 49: 1096 - 1101.

102) Mundo, M. A., Padilla Zakour, O. I and Worobo, R. W. 2004. Growth inhibition of foodborne pathogens and food spoilage organisms by select raw honeys. *International Journal of Food Microbiology,* 97: 1 - 8.

103) Nakajima, Y., Ishibashi, J., Yukuhiro, F., Asaoka, A., Taylor, D and Yamakawa, M. 2003. Antibacterial activity and mechanism of action of tick defensin against Gram-positive bacteria. *Biochimica et Biophysica Acta,* 1624: 125 - 130.

104) Newman, D. J and Cragg, G. M. 2007. Natural products as sources of new drugs over the last 25 years. *Journal of Natural Products,* 70: 461 - 477.

105) Newman, D. J and Cragg, G. M. 2012. Natural products as sources of new drugs over the 30 years from 1981 to 2010. *Journal of Natural Products,* 75: 311 - 335.

106) O'Neill, J. 2014. Antimicrobial resistance: Tackling a crisis for the health and wealth of nation.

107) Oddo, L. P., Piro, R., Bruneau, E., Guyot Declerck, C., Ivanov, T., Piskulova, J., Flamini, C., Lheritier, J., Morlot, M and Russmann, H. 2004. Main European unifloral honeys: descriptive sheets. *Apidologie,* 35: S38 - S81.

108) Orsolic, N., Knezevic, A. H., Sver, L., Terzic, S., Heckenberger, B. K and Basic, I. 2013. Influence of honey bee products on transplantable murine tumours. *Veterinary and Oncology,* 1: 216 - 226.

109) Osho, A and Bello, O. O. 2010. Antimicrobial effect of honey produced by *Apis mellifera* on some common human pathogens. *Asian Journal of Experimental Biology and Science,* 1(4): 875 - 880.

110) Pinho, E., Ferreira, I. C., Barros, L., Carvalho, A. M., Soares, G and Henriques, M. 2014. Antibacterial potential of northeastern Portugal wild plant extracts and respective phenolic compounds. *Biomed Research International,* 81: 45 - 90.

111) Pontes, M., Marques, J. C and Camara, J. S. 2007. Screening of volatile composition from Portuguese multifloral honeys using headspace solid-phase microextraction - gas chromatography-quadrupole mass spectrometry. *Talanta,* 74: 91 - 103.

112) Potts, S. G., Biesmeijer, J. C., Kremen, C., Neumann, P., Schweiger, O and Kunin, W. E. 2010. Global pollinator declines: trends, impacts and drivers. *Trends in Ecology and Evolution,* 25: 345 - 353.

113) Pyrzynska, K and Biesaga, M. 2009. Analysis of phenolic acids and flavonoids in honey. *Trends in Analytical Chemistry,* 28: 893 - 902.

114) Rakhi K., Chute, N. G., Deogade, D and Meghna Kawale. 2010. Antimicrobial activity of Indian honey against clinical isolates. *Asiatic Journal of Biotechnology Resources,* 01: 35 - 38.

115) Ratnieks, F. L. W and Carreck, N. L. 2010. Clarity on Honey Bee Collapse? *Science,* 327: 152 - 153.

116) Sahl, H. G., Pag, U., Bonness, S., Wagner, S., Antcheva, N and Tossi, A. 2005. Mammalian defensins: structures and mechanism of antibiotic activity. *Journal of Leukocyte Biology,* 77: 466 – 475.

117) Sampath Kumar, K. P., Debjit Bhowmik, Chiranjib, Biswajit and M. R. Chandira. 2010. Medicinal uses and health benefits of Honey: An Overview. *Journal of Chemistry and Pharmacy Research,* 2 (1): 385 – 395.

118) Sanchez, V., Baeza, R., Ciappini, C., Zamora M. C and Chirife, J. 2010. Comparison between Karl Fischer and refractometric method for determination of moisture in honey. *Food Control,* 21: 339 - 341.

119) Saranraj, P., Sivasakthi, S and Glaucio Dire Feliciano. 2016. Pharmacology of Honey – A Review. *Advances in Biological Research,* 10 (4): 271 - 289.

120) Sato, T and Miyata, G. 2000. The Nutraceutical Benefit, Part III: Honey. *Nutrition,* 16: 468 - 469.

121) Schmitt, E. K., Moore, C. M., Krastel, P and Petersen, F. 2011. Natural products as catalysts for innovation: a pharmaceutical industry perspective. *Current Opinion in Chemical Biology,* 15: 497 - 504.

122) Silici, S., Sagdic, O and Ekici, L. 2010. Total phenolic content, antiradical, antioxidant and antimicrobial activities of *Rhododendron* honeys. *Food Chemistry,* 121: 238 - 243.

123) Simon, A., Santos, K., Blaser, G., Bode, U and Molan, P. 2009. Medical honey for wound carestill the 'last resort'? *eCAM,* 6: 165 – 173.

124) Singh, S. B and Barrett, J. F. 2006. Empirical antibacterial drug discovery - Foundation in natural products. *Biochemical Pharmacology,* 71: 1006 - 1015.

125) Srisayam, M. and Chantawannakul, P. 2010. Antimicrobial and antioxidant properties of honeys produced by Apis Mellifera in Thailand. *Journal of Apiproduct and Apimedical Science*, 2 (2): 77 - 83.

126) Style, S. 1992. Honey: From Hive to Honeypot. London: Pavilion

127) Subrahmanyam, M. 1991. Topical application of honey in treatment of burns. *Brazilian Journal of Surgery*, 78: 497 – 498.

128) Sumner, L. W., Lei, Z., Nikolau, B. J and Saito, K. 2015. Modern plant metabolomics: advanced natural product gene discoveries, improved technologies, and future prospects. *Natural Product Reports,* 32: 212 - 229.

129) Swellam, T., Miyanaga, N., Onozawa, M., Hattori, K., Kawai, K., Shimazui, T and Akaza, H. 2013. Antineoplastic activity of honey in an experimental bladder cancer implantation model: *in vivo* and *in vitro* studies. *International Journal of Urology*, 10: 213 - 219.

130) Tannahill, R. 1975. Food in History. St Albans: Paladin.

131) Terrab. A., Hernanz, D and Heredia, F. J. 2004. Inductively coupled plasma optical emission spectrometric determination of minerals in thyme honeys and their contribution to geographical discrimination. *Journal of Agriculture and Food Chemistry,* 52: 3441- 3445.

132) Van Herpen, T. W. J. M., Cankar, K., Nogueira, M., Bosch, D., Bouwmeester, H. J and Beekwilder, J. 2010. *Nicotiana benthamiana* as a production platform for artemisinin precursors. *PLoS ONE,* 5: e14222.

133) Visavadia, B., Honeysett, J. D and Martin, H. 2009. Manuka honey dressing: An effective treatment for chronic wound infections. *European Journal of Clinical Microbiology and Infectious Disease*, 28: 339 - 344.

134) Viuda Martos, M., Ruiz Navajas, Y., Fernandez Lopez, J and Perez - Alvarez, J. A. 2008. Functional properties of honey, propolis, and royal jelly. *Journal of Food Science,* 73: R117 - R124.

135) Weston, R. J. 2000. The contribution of catalase and other natural products to the antibacterial activity of honey: A review. *Food Chemistry,* 71: 235 - 239.

136) White, J. W and Subers, M. H. 2013. Studies on honey inhibine, a chemical assay. *Journal of Apiculture Research*, 15: 23 - 28.

137) White, J. W. 1975. Physical characteristics of honey. In: Crane E (ed) Honey, A Comprehensive Survey, Hienemann, London, UK, 207 - 239.

138) WHO. 2014. Antimicrobial resistance: global report on surveillance World Health Organization.

139) Wilson, C. A. 1973. Food and Drink in Britain: From the Stone Age to Recent Times. London: Constable.

140) Wilson, M. B., Spivak, M., Hegeman, A. D., Rendahl, A and Cohen, J. D. 2013. Metabolomics reveals the origins of antimicrobial plant resins collected by honey bees. *PLoS ONE,* 8: e77512.

141) Won, S. R., Li, C. Y., Kim, J. W and Rhee, H. I. 2009. Immunological characterization of honey major protein and its application. *Food Chemistry,* 113: 1334 - 1338.

142) Wooley J. C., Godzik, A and Fredberg, I. 2010. A Primer on Metagenomics. *PLoS Computational Biology,* 6: e1000667.

143) Zappalà, M., Fallico, B., Arena, E and Verzera, A. 2005. Methods for the determination of HMF in honey: A comparison. *Food Control,* 16: 273 - 277.

144) Zumla A. and Lulat A. 1989. Honey - a remedy rediscovered. *Journal of Social Medicine,* 82: 384 - 385.

www.ingramcontent.com/pod-product-compliance
Lightning Source LLC
Chambersburg PA
CBHW081456220526
45466CB00008B/2666